Easy Hikes

CLOSE to
Home

ATLANTA

including
Marietta, Lawrenceville, and Peachtree City

RANDY AND PAM GOLDEN

D1243922

MENASHA RIDGE PRESS
Birmingham, Alabama

This book is meant only as a guide to select trails in the Atlanta area and does not guarantee hiker safety in any way—you hike at your own risk. Neither Menasha Ridge Press nor Randy or Pam Golden is liable for property loss or damage, personal injury, or death that result in any way from accessing or hiking the trails described in the following pages. Please be aware that hikers have been injured in the Atlanta area. Be especially cautious when walking on or near boulders, steep inclines, and drop-offs, and do not attempt to explore terrain that may be beyond your abilities. To help ensure an uneventful hike, please read carefully the introduction to this book, and perhaps get further safety information and guidance from other sources. Familiarize yourself thoroughly with the areas you intend to visit before venturing out. Ask questions, and prepare for the unforeseen. Familiarize yourself with current weather reports, maps of the area you intend to visit, and any relevant park regulations.

Copyright © 2009 Randy and Pam Golden
All rights reserved
Printed in the United States of America
Published by Menasha Ridge Press
Distributed by Publishers Group West
First edition, first printing

ISBN 978-0-89732-726-8

Cover by Scott McGrew
Cover photo by Randy and Pam Golden
Text design by Annie Long
Maps by Randy and Pam Golden, Scott McGrew, and Steve Jones
All interior photos by Randy and Pam Golden

Menasha Ridge Press
P.O. Box 43673
Birmingham, AL 35243
www.menasharidge.com

Contents

About the Authors

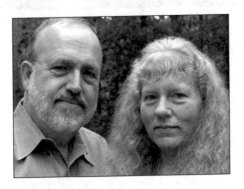

Randy and Pam Golden

Randy and Pam Golden have shared their lifelong love of hiking since they met at college in Florida in 1975. After marrying in 1977, they began hiking across the United States and into Canada. Among their favorite foreign destinations are Puerto Rico's El Yunque and Australia's Dandenong Mountains. They began writing about their adventures on About North Georgia (**www.ngeorgia.com**) in 1995. In 1998 the site's Trails section was spun off into a site of its own, Georgia Trails (**www.georgiatrails.com**).

Introduction

Welcome to *Easy Hikes Close to Home: Atlanta*. This title in the *Easy Hikes* series is organized according to three regions: Atlanta; Atlanta North; and Atlanta South.

Numbered map icons on the inside front cover locate each primary trailhead and are keyed to the table of contents and narrative text for each trail. On the inside back cover, a map legend defines symbols for parking, restrooms, trail features, and other details. Armed with this handy guidebook, you can quickly head out the door and, well, take a hike!

Overview

Mileage shown for each hike corresponds to the total distance from start to finish, for loops, out-and-backs, figure eights, or a combination of shapes. You can shorten or extend some of the hikes with connecting trails.

Trail Maps

Maps for each hike include GPS coordinates. Based on data downloaded from the author's handheld GPS unit and and plotted onto a digital U.S. Geological Survey (USGS) topo map, the coordinates are shown in two formats—as latitude/longitude and as UTM (Universal Transverse Mercator) coordinates.

HIKING ESSENTIALS

Boots should be your footwear of choice. Sport sandals are popular, but they leave much of your foot exposed and vulnerable to hazardous plants, thorns, rocks, and sharp twigs.

When it comes to water, err on the side of excess. Hydrate prior to your hike, carry (and drink) six ounces of water for every mile you plan to hike, and hydrate after the hike. Pack along a couple of small bottles on even short hikes. You may decide to linger, or take an alternate route and extend your time outdoors.

Always plan for unpredictable scenarios by carrying these items, in addition to water:

Map

Compass

Basic first-aid supplies, such as Band-Aids and aspirin

Knife

Windproof matches or a lighter and fire starter

Snacks

Flashlight with extra batteries

Rain protection and a sweater or windbreaker, even in warm weather

Sun protection

Insect repellent

Whistle

GENERAL TIPS

The whole point of your outing is to enjoy nature, fresh air, and exercise. Here are a few tips to enhance your excursion:

- Avoid weekends and traditional holidays if possible; otherwise, go early in the morning. Trails that are packed in the summer are often clear during the colder months and during rainy times (but never hike during a thunderstorm).

- Before you hit the trail, double-check your map, and don't set out on the trail until you have the information you need.

- Once on the trail, be careful at overlooks, stay back from the edge of outcrops, and be absolutely sure of your footing wherever you are.

- Hike on open trails only. Respect trail and road closures, avoid trespassing on private land, and obtain permits if required. Leave gates as you found them or as marked.

- Stay on the existing trail, and avoid any littering.

- When hiking with children, use common sense to judge a child's capacity to hike a particular trail, and expect that the child may tire and need to be carried. Make sure children are adequately clothed for the weather, have proper shoes, and are protected from the sun with sunscreen. Kids dehydrate quickly, so make sure you have plenty of fluids for everyone.

- Take your time along the trails, whether you are doing one of this guide's short hikes or hours-long treks. In other words: Don't miss the trees for the forest. You may finish some of the "hike times" long before or after that suggested in the Overview box. A short-distance hike with a lot of up-and-downs may take more time and energy than a longer, flatter hike.

- Participate in some online wildlife observation counts. Cornell Lab of Ornithology operates **www.ebird.org** where you can login for free and submit bird lists or find out what's being seen at some of the area's birding hot spots. A similar count is being done for butterflies at **www.wisconsinbutterflies.org/butterflies/sightings.**

- Never spook animals. An unannounced approach, a sudden movement, or a loud noise startles most animals, and a surprised animal can be dangerous. Give them plenty of space.

- Be courteous to others you encounter on the trails.

- Look up! Keep an eye out for standing dead trees and storm-damaged living trees with loose or broken limbs that can fall at any time.

- Know your ability, and carry necessary supplies for changes in weather or other conditions.

TRAIL RECOMMENDATIONS

BUSY HIKES

1 Atlanta Ramble
3 Grant Park Loop (includes Zoo Atlanta)
13 McDaniel Farm Park Trail

HIKES FEATURING WATERFALLS

16 Cochran Mill Trail

HIKES FEATURING WILDFLOWERS

6 Reynolds Nature Preserve
7 Chattahoochee Nature Center Trail
13 McDaniel Farm Park Trail
19 Piedmont National Wildlife Refuge Trails

HIKES GOOD FOR CHILDREN

2 Big Trees Preserve Trail
3 Grant Park Loop (includes Zoo Atlanta)
7 Chattahoochee Nature Center Trail
13 McDaniel Farm Park Trail

HIKES GOOD FOR SOLITUDE

17 Ocmulgee River Trail
19 Piedmont National Wildlife Refuge Trails

HIKES GOOD FOR WILDLIFE VIEWING

7 Chattahoochee Nature Center Trail
19 Piedmont National Wildlife Refuge Trails

HIKES LESS THAN 3 MILES

2 Big Trees Preserve Trail
4 Johnson Ferry Trail
6 Reynolds Nature Preserve
7 Chattahoochee Nature Center Trail
11 Bowman's Island Trail
13 McDaniel Farm Park Trail
15 Starrs Mill Trail
16 Cochran Mill Trail
18 Panola Mountain Trail

HIKES 3 TO 6 MILES

1 Atlanta Ramble
3 Grant Park Loop (includes Zoo Atlanta)
5 Powers Landing Trail
8 Cheatham Hill Trail
9 Heritage Park Trail
10 Homestead Trail
12 Jones Bridge Trail
14 Stone Mountain Loop
17 Ocmulgee River Trail
19 Piedmont National Wildlife Refuge Trails

HISTORIC TRAILS

8 Cheatham Hill Trail
9 Heritage Park Trail
12 Jones Bridge Trail
13 McDaniel Farm Park Trail
16 Cochran Mill Trail

LAKE HIKES

7 Chattahoochee Nature Center Trail
10 Homestead Trail

TRAILS GOOD FOR RUNNERS

3 Grant Park Loop (includes Zoo Atlanta)
10 Homestead Trail
13 McDaniel Farm Park Trail

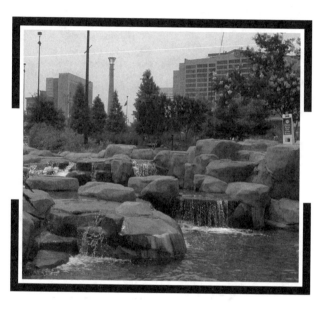

Atlanta

01 *Atlanta Ramble*

■ OVERVIEW

LENGTH: 5.4 miles	**ACCESS:** Open year-round
CONFIGURATION: Loop	**MAPS:** Atlanta Convention and Visitors Bureau; Atlanta Chamber of Commerce; USGS Southwest Atlanta, Northwest Atlanta
SCENERY: Urban scenes, including high-rise buildings	
EXPOSURE: Full sun	
TRAFFIC: Heavy	**FACILITIES:** All necessary facilities found throughout
TRAIL SURFACE: Concrete sidewalks	**SPECIAL COMMENTS:** Underground Atlanta has a number of excellent restaurants.
HIKING TIME: 5 hours	

■ SNAPSHOT

From Ted Turner Field, this hike visits the capitol dome, Underground Atlanta, Georgia Dome, Philips Arena, CNN Center, Centennial Park, the Georgia Aquarium, and the World of Coca-Cola.

■ CLOSE-UP

This hike begins in the parking lot opposite Turner Field, at the site of the original Atlanta–Fulton County Stadium. From the parking lot is a great view of downtown Atlanta and the Olympic flame. Turner Field was built to house the Olympics and then converted into a baseball field to replace the aging Fulton County Stadium. A plaque commemorates the most historic moment that occurred at the original structure—Henry (Hank) Aaron's 715th home run, which he hit on April 6, 1974, breaking Babe Ruth's long-standing record.

Turn around, cross Georgia Avenue, and enter Turner Field at the black-iron gates. Purchase tickets for the tour in the box office, and view the Braves Hall of Fame Museum before the tour. In addition to a World Series trophy, they have a railroad car

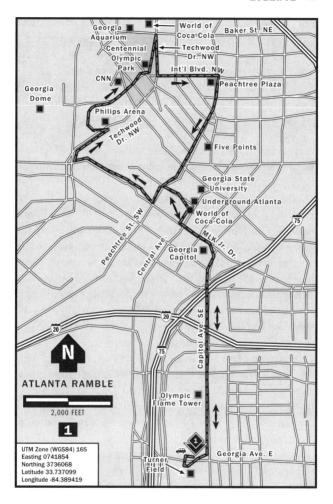

the Braves used in the 1950s and a display on the various fields in which the Braves have played. The tour visits the Braves dugout and bullpen, and takes you next to the ball field and then into the locker room. Off-season hours are Monday through Saturday from 10 a.m. to 2 p.m. Beginning April 1, tours are offered Monday through Saturday from 9 a.m. to 3 p.m. and Sunday from 1 p.m. to 3 p.m. On game days, tours are offered from 9 a.m. to noon. Tours start on the hour and last about an hour.

When exiting Turner Field, turn right on Georgia Avenue, then turn left on Henry Aaron Drive, crossing under the Olympic rings and passing the flame on your left. At 0.9 miles the Georgia State Capitol is on the left. Inside the building, which is open from 8 a.m. to 5 p.m. Monday through Friday, is a large number of displays about the cultural and natural history of Georgia, including Georgia's role in the civil rights movement. On the grounds are statues of some fairly well-known Georgia politicians, including Jimmy Carter, Richard B. Russell, and John B. Gordon, among others. After looping around the grounds, return to MLK Jr. Drive, cross the street, and turn left. On the corner of MLK Jr. Drive and Washington Street, notice the statue to the working dogs whose heroism saved many lives during the terrorist attacks on the World Trade Center in New York City. After crossing Central Avenue, you will see the old World of Coca-Cola building on the right, which marks the start of Underground Atlanta.

As you leave the area, look across an open area for a mural of whales. Below that is the 1869 Atlanta Depot, now an upscale restaurant. When this freight depot was completed, it was the tallest building in Atlanta, but a 1935 fire destroyed the second floor. Turn left just before the depot and enter Underground Atlanta.

A potpourri of shops, restaurants, and nightclubs, the three-level Underground Atlanta is a vast underground city within a city. Directly in front of you is an information kiosk and many restaurants. Underground Atlanta was created at the start of the 20th century, when the population of Atlanta had soared to 200,000 people. Crossing the tracks through downtown had become a major traffic snarl, so the government added an iron bridge to speed up traffic. In 1929 the iron bridge was converted into a concrete viaduct, and businesses moved their storefronts to the second story of the buildings.

At the end of the food court, turn left and take the escalator to Kenny's Alley. Turn left again and stroll down Upper Alabama Street to Peachtree Street just south of Five Points. Turn left on Peachtree and right on MLK Jr. Drive, and walk 0.4 miles to Centennial Olympic Park Drive. Directly before you is the white-roofed, red-sided Georgia Dome, home of the Atlanta Falcons. Turn right on Centennial Drive and continue past the MARTA (Metropolitan Atlanta Rapid Transit Authority) station until you are standing directly in front of Philips Arena. This new site is home to the Atlanta Hawks and the Atlanta Thrashers. Note the word "Atlanta" spelled in white letters in the front of the building. Turn around and walk back to the first road on the right, and turn right.

At the end of this road is one of the three massive buildings that compose the Georgia World Congress Center (GWCC). Built on the site of the old Atlanta roundhouse, the Congress Center is home to hundreds of industry shows a year. It was this area that was heavily damaged in the 2008 Atlanta tornado. Turn right and continue down International Boulevard, passing the CNN Center and Omni Hotel on the right and the Atlanta Chamber of Commerce on the left.

You are now in the center of Atlanta's Centennial Olympic Park. Designed by EDAW and built by Beers-Russell, the park features the Fountain of Rings, the Great Lawn, the Water Gardens, and five unique "quilt plazas" telling the story of the Atlanta Olympics; the Quilt of Remembrance was designed to tell the story of the bombing that killed 2 people and injured 118 more in the park. After viewing the Fountain of Rings on the right, turn left and walk to the reflecting pool. With the pool on your immediate left, there is a trail almost directly in front of you. This leads to the Water Gardens, our favorite part of the park. Follow the path 0.1 mile to reach the Georgia Agricultural Plaza on Baker Street. The Georgia Aquarium, the world's largest aquarium, opened in November 2005. Within the aquarium are five areas, including Cold Water Quest, Georgia Explorer, Ocean Voyager, River Scout, and Tropical Diver.

The World of Coca-Cola, next to the aquarium, is a multi-media presentation designed to educate and fascinate visitors. Exhibiting early print ads, modern TV commercials, and everything in between, the displays take visitors through the development of Coca-Cola's image and products. Turn right on Baker Street, right again on Centennial Olympic Park Drive, and then left on Andrew Young International Boulevard. On the left are the Gift Mart and the Merchandise Mart. On the right is the impressive 72-story Westin Peachtree Plaza, a fixture of the Atlanta skyline and home of the most exciting elevator ride in the southeastern United States. The ride climbs the outside of the building, affording a complete view of the city. At the top, the Sundial restaurant and lounge makes a complete revolution every hour.

Turn right (south) on Peachtree Street, Atlanta's main boulevard. When the Fulton County Library comes into view just south of Carnegie Way, you are entering the oldest area of Atlanta, known as the Fairlie-Poplar District. It was here that the first residential homes were constructed, to be replaced by commercial structures after the Civil War. Today the district is an amalgam of old and new buildings blending together almost seamlessly. Continuing south on Peachtree Street, you'll see Woodruff Park on the left. Watch for the Coca-Cola Spectacular, followed by Five Points, created by the intersection of Peachtree, Marietta, and Decatur streets and Edgewood Avenue. Continue south on Peachtree two more blocks and turn left into Underground Atlanta. From this point, retrace your steps to Turner Field.

■ MORE FUN

The APEX Museum on Auburn Avenue looks at the history of African Americans in the city of Atlanta. Fittingly situated on Auburn Avenue, the economic and cultural center for African Americans when Atlanta was segregated, the museum explores the economic and cultural rise of the Sweet Auburn District.

Turn left two blocks after Carnegie Way on Auburn Avenue. The museum is two blocks down on your right and is open in February and from June through August only, Tuesday through Saturday, from 10 a.m. to 5 p.m., and Sunday, from 1 p.m. to 5 p.m.

■ TO THE TRAILHEAD

Take Interstate 75/85 South to Exit 246 (Fulton Street). At the end of the ramp, turn left and travel 0.2 miles. Turn right on Hank Aaron Drive (also known as Capitol Avenue). At Georgia Avenue turn right again and enter the Green Lot on the right.

02 *Big Trees Preserve Trail*

■ OVERVIEW

LENGTH: 1.2 miles	**MAPS:** Available at stand at trailhead. Look for a stapled, multi-page hand-out—the map is on the last page; USGS Chamblee.
CONFIGURATION: Loop	
SCENERY: Streamside and water-shed views of Powers Branch	
EXPOSURE: Mostly shaded	**FACILITIES:** None
TRAFFIC: Moderate	**SPECIAL COMMENTS:** Big Trees Trail parking can be crowded because it is also the parking lot for the North Fulton Annex. Dogs must be leashed at all times and cleaned up after; this is strictly enforced.
TRAIL SURFACE: Packed dirt	
HIKING TIME: 45 minutes	
ACCESS: Open year-round, dawn–dusk	

■ SNAPSHOT

Big Trees has multiple loops and straight-line trails that can be combined for a wide variety of hikes. A 300-foot climb on the Backcountry Loop is so well done it seems effortless.

■ CLOSE-UP

The John Ripley Forbes Big Trees Forest Preserve was created and is managed by the Southeast Land Preservation Trust in

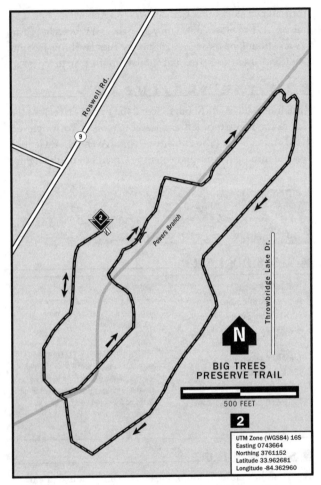

Roswell Rd.

9

Powers Branch

Throwbridge Lake Dr.

N

BIG TREES
PRESERVE TRAIL

500 FEET

2

UTM Zone (WGS84) 16S
Easting 0743664
Northing 3761152
Latitude 33.962681
Longitude -84.362960

partnership with both Fulton County and the state of Georgia, which technically own the land. At 30 acres, it is one of the largest undeveloped tracts in the city of Sandy Springs, north of Atlanta. It is named in honor of John Ripley Forbes, a naturalist who worked extensively with local governments nationwide to preserve land. Mr. Forbes's legacy in Atlanta includes both the Fernbank Museum and the Chattahoochee Nature Center.

From the trailhead, the paved path begins an easy descent into the Powers Branch watershed. Immediately visible to the right is the pre-1902 roadbed of Roswell Road, a major Atlanta-area road that permitted Roswell-area mills access to the railhead in Atlanta and served every town north of the Chattahoochee. The Big Trees Loop splits at a marked intersection right up ahead. Continue straight on the split-rail fence–lined, chip-covered path as the paved trail bears left. As it descends, Big Trees Loop almost imperceptibly joins the old roadbed.

Bear right on Powers Branch Trail at 0.1 mile as Big Trees Loop Trail continues around to the left. As you descend to the creek, Beech Hollow Trail heads right, quickly falling to a loop around a massive American beech. At the bottom is a scenic side view of the creek near the culvert that carries the stream under the present-day Roswell Road. There are tree-stump seats, if you want to spend a few minutes in quiet reflection. As you return to Powers Branch Trail, turn right and descend to a 90-degree left-hand turn as the pathway joins Powers Branch. Continue straight when the Backcountry Connector heads right a few steps after the turn.

Over the next 0.2 miles, the trail climbs about 100 feet on an easy hike into the Powers Branch Watershed. The path twice crosses the stream: once on a wooden bridge, then on an interesting "rock hop"—a planned, raised rock path through the water. The stream runs through a concealed culvert underneath a large rock in the center. The kids will love this!

Just over 0.5 miles into the hike, the boulders get larger, but even an untrained eye can tell that the formation is not natural. On the left as you enter the area is an old road grade that disappears into the modern embankment of the North Fulton Annex. A small cascade in the river makes a pretty photograph, but the telltale drill hole gives away the secret—the falls are man-made. Just past the falls, Powers Branch Trail ends as Spring Hollow Trail turns right, crosses an unrailed bridge over the creek, and rises to the Backcountry Connector. Make a hard left at the end of the brief Spring Hollow Trail.

The Backcountry Connector continues to climb, paralleling the creek. As apartments come into view straight ahead, look down to the left. The creek is now 60 feet below the footpath. A few steps later the trail begins an easy double switch to climb to its highest point, just a few feet after the second switchback. From this point, the treadway begins an easy descent through a second-growth hardwood forest comprised of white and post oak and American beech interspersed with native azalea.

As the hike approaches 1 mile, the footpath begins an easy curve to the right. At the end of the curve, the path runs adjacent to the grade of the Bull Sluice Railroad, built in 1902 to move material to the site of Morgan Falls Dam, one of the earliest hydroelectric projects in the state. After work on the dam was completed, the railbed was abandoned. At 1 mile, a path to the left crosses a bridge and makes a switchback ascent to a patio adjacent to a Ford dealership. A small portion of this path actually runs on the level grade of the old railroad bed.

Just past this bridge is the left turn onto the short Backwoods Connector Trail. Cross a wooden bridge, turn to the left on Powers Branch Trail, and follow the path around to the right to return to the trailhead.

■ MORE FUN

Heritage Sandy Springs is an interpreted farmhouse and museum and the site of the five freshwater springs for which the city is named. The park, on Sandy Springs Circle just off Hammond Drive, is open daily from dawn to dusk.

■ TO THE TRAILHEAD

Take GA 400 North to Exit 6, Northridge Road. Circle around and turn right at the end of the exit ramp. In 0.4 miles turn left on GA 9, known locally as Roswell Road. Continue south 1.4

miles to the North Fulton Annex, just past Morgan Falls Dam Road on the right. Turn left into the second (south) parking lot and look for the trailhead directly in front of you on the right.

03   *Grant Park Loop (includes Zoo Atlanta)*

■ OVERVIEW

LENGTH: 3.1 miles	**HIKING TIME:** 3.5 hours
CONFIGURATION: Loop	**ACCESS:** Open year-round
SCENERY: Well-kept, historic park with huge trees in a generally upscale downtown area	**MAPS:** Available at Zoo Atlanta; USGS Southeast Atlanta
EXPOSURE: Partial shade to full sun	**FACILITIES:** Restrooms, playgrounds, Civil War museum and Cyclorama; Zoo Atlanta
TRAFFIC: Heavy, especially in Zoo Atlanta	**SPECIAL COMMENTS:** This is a great family hike, featuring the zoo, playgrounds, and fast food.
TRAIL SURFACE: Almost entirely paved	

■ SNAPSHOT

Grant Park Loop visits the 1880s-era green space that was the centerpiece of a development of wealthy homes. The park also houses Zoo Atlanta, which features animals living in near-native habitats.

■ CLOSE-UP

Each year, more than 2 million people visit Grant Park to see the world-class Zoo Atlanta, view a three-dimensional re-creation of the Civil War's Battle of Atlanta, see downtown from a Civil War fort, or just relax in the green space created by Lemuel Grant, for whom the park is named. Grant, who moved to Georgia from Maine in the late 1830s, was one of Atlanta's first citizens. He designed a series of defenses around the city that

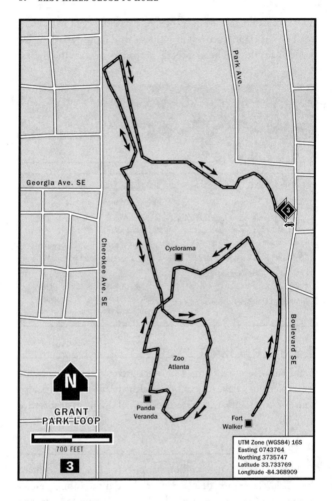

helped the Confederate army defend the city against a Union onslaught. After the Civil War, Grant played a key role in Atlanta's revitalization. He began organizing the park in 1881 and donated it to the city of Atlanta in 1883.

Grant Park has always been open to both blacks and whites, an unusual occurrence in the segregated South. Even the zoo was integrated—sort of. The Atlanta attraction regularly had "black-only" days. In 1921 Atlanta added the Cyclorama, a building to house the *Battle of Atlanta* painting. It also moved the Civil War locomotive The Texas, which had sat exposed in Grant Park, inside the building.

On a paved road across from the first lane of parking (the lane nearest the entrance), walk through four white posts underneath the spreading crowns of a group of old-growth post oaks. As the paved road begins an easy curve to the left, a side road leaves to the right. The road then curves back to the right as it heads toward a hill with a gazebo on top. Continue to bear right as the road splits in front of the gazebo, and you will reach a five-road intersection. Bear left on a road that descends then curves right. At 0.3 miles turn right. A few steps down this paved road is a small playground up on the right. As the road begins to rise, turn right on a paved road; immediately on the left is the massive stone fountain and a park entrance that was added in the early 1900s. Circle the structure, which is being restored by the Grant Park Conservancy, then make the first left and climb a short way to street level. Two roads enter Grant Park at 45-degree angles from Cherokee Avenue, which forms the eastern boundary of the park. This is a popular place to take a picture, but plan to get there later in the day and shoot from the far side of street. Continue to circle to the left, descending on the other side of the entrance.

At the end of the road, turn right at the T-intersection and climb to Cherokee Avenue for more views of both Grant Park and the surrounding neighborhood. The area is being rejuvenated thanks to low-interest loans from the city. Turn left and walk on the sidewalk, making the next left to head back into the park. As this road descends, it curves right, crossing a culvert on a concrete bridge. Just past the bridge is Constitution Spring, which was once one of five mineral springs within the park. A stone bridge sits in a tree-lined open field on the left of the road at 0.9 miles.

The road curves around to the left, coming out at the entrance to Zoo Atlanta. This nationally recognized zoo allows species to roam freely in specially designed areas intended to mimic the animal's natural habitat. Back in 1984, Atlantans discovered that the Metropolitan Zoo had been named one of the ten worst in the country. Some spoke of closing the zoo and returning Willie B., a silverback gorilla at the center of the controversy, to his home in Cameroon. Rather than give up, Atlanta hired a new director for the attraction, Terry Maples, who began the arduous task of completely rebuilding the zoo.

Stunning pink flamingos greet visitors just inside the entrance. Close by are elephants, the critically endangered black rhino, and a lion; then it's off to the Ford African Rain Forest. Willie B. died in 2000, but his offspring carry on the strong tradition of the rain forest in Atlanta, where multiple viewing sites allow glimpses into the lives of these stoic creatures. At the end of the rain forest, there are other animals and reptiles, but follow the path on the left just past a food kiosk to the panda exhibit for a one-of-a-kind treat.

Considered the symbol of peace in its homeland of China, the giant panda is a black-and-white fur-bearing mammal with markings similar to those of the raccoon, but DNA testing has proven it is in the bear family. Lun-Lun and Yang-Yang arrived at Zoo Atlanta in November 1999 for a ten-year stay and immediately became stars in the animal-oriented attraction. The endangered pandas occasionally play together, but mostly they eat bamboo in separate sections of their environment. A line forms quickly at this exhibit, so plan a 20- to 30-minute wait.

As you leave, the Panda Veranda is on the left, complete with picnic tables and a McDonald's. If you don't need a break, continue straight ahead to view the zoo's two Sumatran tigers. One of a handful of zoos with a captive breeding program, Zoo Atlanta is active in the fight to save this nearly extinct species.

Fewer that 400 Sumatran tigers are known to exist in the wild or in captivity. As you exit the tiger exhibit, follow the road that bears left toward the Ford Pavilion, then follow the path to the right and turn right into the Kids Zone. Immediately after the turn is a marked railroad crossing for a train that young children can ride. Kids can get close to animals in the petting zoo and see kangaroos, but for our favorite exhibit, turn left at Base Camp Discovery and follow the path around to the left. Here, tortoises take their time exploring the habitat created by the zoo. These mammoth prehistoric beasts are fun to watch as they eat, sleep, or walk.

As you leave the Kids Zone, turn right; the exit is almost directly in front of you. After passing through the booths, on the left is the Cyclorama. Built in 1921, it houses a three-dimensional painting in the round, *The Battle of Atlanta,* and a Civil War museum featuring The Texas, one of the locomotives involved in the Great Locomotive Chase.

After viewing the museum and the painting, exit and turn right. Turn right again on the first concrete path to wind back to the parking lot. Once in the parking lot, turn right and walk to the southern end of the lot. Follow the road around to the left and turn right on the paved path at the end of the second lane of parking. This path winds to Fort Walker, an earthen outpost along the defenses constructed by Grant. It is one of the few remaining intact Civil War sites in the Atlanta metropolitan area. From the top of the hill there is a good view of the downtown skyline. Return to the parking lot using the same path you followed to Fort Walker.

■ TO THE TRAILHEAD

Take I-20 East to Exit 59A (Boulevard). At the end of the ramp, turn right and travel 0.4 miles to the parking lot on the right. If the parking lot is full, continue south on Boulevard to Atlanta Avenue; turn right, right again on Cherokee Street, and right into a second parking lot.

■ OVERVIEW

LENGTH: 2.1 miles

CONFIGURATION: Balloon

SCENERY: There are some long-distance views of the Chattahoochee River and a forested wetland in the river's floodplain.

EXPOSURE: Full sun at the start and end of the hike, mostly shaded for the rest

TRAFFIC: Light

TRAIL SURFACE: Compact soil

HIKING TIME: 1 hour

ACCESS: Year-round, dawn–dusk

MAPS: Map stands are located on the trail throughout the hike, additional map copies are available from the Chattahoochee River National Recreation Area (CRNRA) main office at Island Ford (see separate listing), or visit them online at www.nps.gov/chat; USGS Sandy Springs

FACILITIES: None

SPECIAL COMMENTS: A National Park Service (NPS) map indicates that seasonal restrooms are available, but this is wrong.

■ SNAPSHOT

This trail explores a floodplain of the Chattahoochee River, including a forested wetland, then joins "the Hooch" for a hike along its riverbank.

■ CLOSE-UP

For more than 20 years, the Chattahoochee Outdoor Center was the summer fun capital for rafting enthusiasts in Atlanta. Each weekend thousands of people would visit the center, located at this hike's trailhead, and take a leisurely float down the Chattahoochee River to one of two takeouts farther south. They closed in 2002 when the number of rafters dropped off after the National Park Service began posting E. coli levels (an indication of pollution) at Johnson Ferry.

From the kiosk at the trailhead, follow the road to descend to a plain that was the parking lot for the Outdoor Center. The road soon changes from pavement to gravel and continues

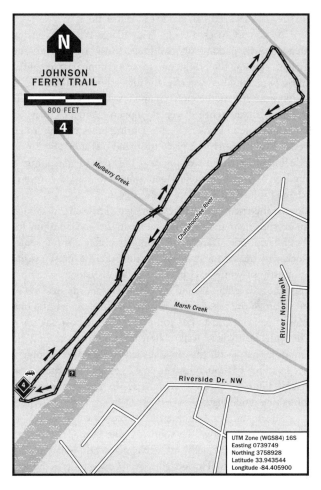

straight ahead. On your right is the return trail for the loop. Once clear of vegetation, the parking lot is in the early stages of natural reclamation. Black-eyed Susans and goldenrod abound in this full-sun portion of Johnson Ferry Trail. Look for the vestiges of humans—an overgrown picnic table here and there, an old tire, or a decayed sign giving exit instructions.

As you approach a bridge with a large Wildlife Viewing Area sign, the parking-lot road loops to the right. Continue straight, crossing the bridge, and make an immediate left at 0.3 miles. Three hundred feet after the turn, a boardwalk first takes you across a stream then into an up-close view of the wetlands of the Chattahoochee River floodplain. Wetlands play an important role in a river's health. During times of high water, wetlands give the river a place to spread out and slow down, reducing downstream erosion. Also, they provide habitat for a number of small mammals and waterfowl and a breeding ground for insects, which the river fish eat.

At the end of the bridge, turn right. The wetlands, which are on your right and slightly lower than the trail, continue for about half a mile. They are occasionally visible but frequently blocked by trees along its edges. On this hike, the forest is made up mostly of white oak, beech, and an occasional sycamore tree. The area in and around the wetlands is mostly shaded.

Part of the hike is on a historic roadbed, which the trail joins at 0.6 miles, just after you pass two large post oak trees. The wide, nearly level walk is away from traffic noise, and the sounds of nature fill the air: a distant woodpecker tapping a tree in search of food, birds chirping to establish territory, and playful squirrels loudly crunching leaves and sounding like something much bigger.

Shortly after joining the road, a blowdown of some Virginia pine, courtesy of the southern pine beetle, requires an easy walk-around. Finally, at 1 mile, a recently updated map indicates that the trail turns right. Several other trails in the area drew our attention—one ended at the Chattahoochee River National Recreation Area (CRNRA) property line (marked by double red rings around trees), and the other two ended at a small stream.

Reaching the bank of the Chattahoochee River at 1.2 miles, the pathway makes another hard right, turning to follow the river back to the trailhead. Mostly shaded during this portion of the hike, Johnson Ferry Trail occasionally breaks into full sun for brief periods. When the trail is adjacent to the riverbank, there are some good long-distance river views. There is also a repetitive pattern on the trail: As it approaches each of the Chattahoochee River tributaries, the trail turns right, goes inland about 200 feet to a power-line opening, turns left to cross a bridge, and then turns left again to return to the river. After turning inland the third time, the trail crosses the bridge at the start of the loop, and you are once again in the Chattahoochee Outdoor Center parking lot.

Continue straight until you see the parking-lot road loop to the left. In the distance, almost straight ahead, is the brown fort-like building that used to house the center. As you approach the building, you'll see a narrow trail to the left at 1.9 miles. This takes you down to a Chattahoochee River access ramp that rafters and kayakers occasionally use. As of October 2004, the National Park Service no longer posts water-quality levels at the ramp because of a lack of funding for the project. From the ramp, turn around and face the Outdoor Center building. Walk up the ramp to the end of the cement, and turn left on a wide trail that swings around to the parking lot. Turn left and climb the paved road to the trailhead kiosk.

■ TO THE TRAILHEAD

Take I-285 West to Exit 24, Riverside Drive. At the end of the ramp, turn right. Travel 2.1 miles north on Riverside to Johnson Ferry Road. Turn left at the light, cross the Chattahoochee River, and make an immediate right into the parking lot for the Johnson Ferry North Unit of the CRNRA. Look for a brown kiosk in the center of the north side of the parking lot (opposite the entrance).

05 Powers Landing Trail

■ OVERVIEW

LENGTH: 2.3 miles	**HIKING TIME:** 1.5 hours
CONFIGURATION: Loop	**ACCESS:** Year-round, dawn–dusk
SCENERY: Historic home site, scenic views of the Chattahoochee River	**MAPS:** USGS Sandy Springs
EXPOSURE: Mostly shaded	**FACILITIES:** Restrooms
TRAFFIC: Moderate	**SPECIAL COMMENTS:** Fishing is popular here, with anglers reporting some good brown and rainbow trout and shoal bass.
TRAIL SURFACE: Compact soil and historic roadbed	

■ SNAPSHOT

This trail explores Powers Island in the Chattahoochee River and then follows the floodplain of the river to a wonderful cove in the watershed. As you return to the trailhead, the path offers scenic views of the river.

■ CLOSE-UP

In 1819 the Cherokee signed a treaty with the United States that used this section of the Chattahoochee River to define the eastern boundary of this independent Native American nation. James Powers established a homestead and a ferry here in 1831. The Cherokee and local settlers gave Powers, who was a gunsmith as well as manager of the ferry and blacksmith shop, a brisk business repairing their weapons. When the Land Lottery of 1832 gave the Cherokee Nation away to settlers from Georgia, Powers moved west across the Chattahoochee River in 1833, to Vinings, in the newly formed Cobb County. He continued to oversee the ferry's operation. In 1903 the ferry was replaced by a bridge, near where the present-day I-285 bridge crosses the river.

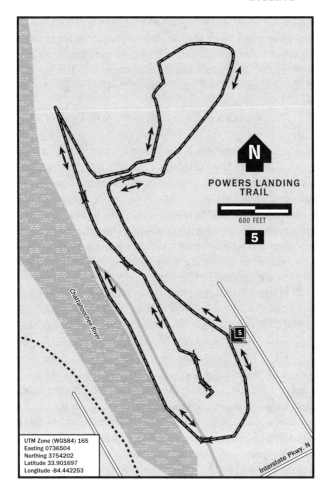

POWERS LANDING
TRAIL

N

600 FEET

5

Chattahoochee River

5

UTM Zone (WGS84) 16S
Easting 0736504
Northing 3754202
Latitude 33.901697
Longitude -84.442253

Interstate Pkwy. N

Circle the brown Chattahoochee Outdoor Center, which
has been closed since 2002, to reach an iron bridge with wooden
slats that connects to Powers Island. Kayaks frequently run the
course between the riverbank and the island. After crossing the
bridge, join the footpath, which bears right, passing a canoe

and kayak launch on the right, and then curves back to the left and crosses the narrow island. When you come to a second launch site, on the windward side of the island, the view of the river opens up. Across the Chattahoochee is the popular Cochran Shoals walking trail. Descend the steps for good views up and down the river.

Turn around and climb back to the path, heading left at the end of the split-rail fence onto a compact dirt trail that follows near the riverbank. Passing through a mostly hardwood forest filled with large oak trees, especially close to the shore, the level treadway runs near the riverbank most of the way to the north end of the island. As you near your destination, the footpath heads inland to cross a small creek in an area of pine blowdown. Finally coming to a wide channel between two islands, this is where the trail ends today. Many years ago this channel did not exist, and it was possible to follow the trail to a deck on the north end of the island.

Return to the start of this trail and turn left. There are two entrances to the loop, but look for the one in the far right-hand corner of the parking lot. Beginning as a wide, level roadway, the pathway comes into a pine blowdown at 0.9 miles. After the blowdown, long poison-ivy vines scale large oak trees, and American beech trees abound. After you cross a culverted creek, the footpath reaches a three-way intersection at 1.1 miles. Turn right and begin climbing a narrower trail. On the left is a woodland stream. After you cross a wooden bridge over a tributary, the trail curves right, climbs a set of stairs, and swings left. As you approach a stone wall, ascend to a small level field that was once a homestead.

On the far side of the homestead is an old roadbed that was once a driveway. At 1.3 miles the roadbed heads right as the trail continues to climb to a ridgetop. As a second trail heads off to the right, the footpath veers left and begins to climb to an unnamed knoll. From there, the path returns to the woodland stream, now on your left. As the trail descends, the rock outcroppings increase, and you can see wildflowers. After a set of wooden steps, the trail returns to the main path in the Chattahoochee floodplain. Turn right, continue to the next map stand, and turn right again.

Back on a gravel road, watch for a heavily damaged deck on the island just off the riverbank. The Powers Island portion of the hike once came this far north, but the changing currents of the Chattahoochee have made it impossible to reach the deck. The park ends in an area of large, poison ivy–covered trees. Turn around, return to the map stand, and continue along the bank of the Chattahoochee River by bearing right.

On the left, at 2.1 miles into the hike, a lone chimney rises, the building that accompanied it long gone. Feel free to explore the area, but watch out for small animals. Return to the path and follow the riverbank back to your car.

■ MORE FUN

This is a great Sunday hike because of Ray's On the River Sunday brunch. This upscale Atlanta eatery has been wowing diners for many years, and for good reason. The food is excellent, and the cost is reasonable. As you leave the parking lot, turn right on Interstate North Parkway and make a left at the first light, onto Powers Ferry Road. Go under I-285 and turn left at the light, also Powers Ferry Road. After you cross the Chattahoochee River, you'll see Ray's in an industrial park; take the first driveway on the right.

■ TO THE TRAILHEAD

Take I-285 West from GA 400 to Exit 22, Northside Drive/New Northside Drive/Powers Ferry Road. As you come off the ramp, bear right on Interstate Parkway North, which curves left. Follow this 0.8 miles and turn right into the parking area just before the Chattahoochee River.

■ OVERVIEW

LENGTH: 1.8 miles	**ACCESS:** Open year-round
CONFIGURATION: Loop	**MAPS:** Available at the trailhead kiosk; USGS Jonesboro
SCENERY: Multiple lakeshore views, forested wetlands, and a 17-foot-circumference white oak that was felled by a storm	**FACILITIES:** Nature center with native animals, restrooms, picnic areas
EXPOSURE: Mostly shaded, except in the vicinity of lakes and dam, where it is sometimes in full sun	**SPECIAL COMMENTS:** There are many chances to see smaller animals, including turtles, tortoises, and a family of beavers, within the park. The nature center is open weekdays, 8:30 a.m.–5:30 p.m., and on the first Saturday of the month, 9 a.m.–1 p.m.
TRAFFIC: Light	
TRAIL SURFACE: Compact soil	
HIKING TIME: 1 hour	

■ SNAPSHOT

Reynolds Preserve, with more than 4 miles of well-made hiking trails, offers an excellent family hike.

■ CLOSE-UP

William H. Reynolds Memorial Nature Preserve is built on the estate of William Huie Reynolds, a county judge who donated 130 acres of land to Clayton County to preserve both forest and wetlands for future generations. The preserve's board of trustees and the county have purchased another 16 acres of adjoining land that was once owned by Judge Reynolds for preservation. Within the boundaries of the park are the Reynolds home, a barn, other outbuildings, a number of ponds and wetlands, a large area of forested hills, and a nature center.

From the trailhead kiosk at the north end of the parking area, follow the paved trail through a mostly pine forest to reach the nature center. Among the pines within the preserve are lob-

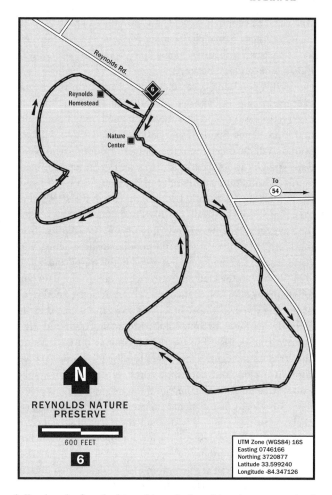

Reynolds Rd.

6

Reynolds
Homestead

Nature
Center

To
54

N

**REYNOLDS NATURE
PRESERVE**

600 FEET

6

UTM Zone (WGS84) 16S
Easting 0746166
Northing 3720877
Latitude 33.599240
Longitude -84.347126

lolly, shortleaf, and white, although the white pines we noticed
were all immature. Almost immediately on the right is the trail
back from the Reynolds home. Continue toward the nature
center. Inside are a number of interesting exhibits, including
small amphibians and reptiles and an active honeybee hive. As

you leave the center, turn right and continue to a paved, wheel-chair-accessible native plant garden adjacent to the nature center. The garden features plants like American beautyberry, Indian pink, and red buckeye.

Wide, level, and covered in mulch, Brookside Trail begins after the brick-paved native plant garden at a marked three-way intersection at 0.1 mile. It is the first named trail in our multi-trail loop. Three hundred feet past this intersection, Hickory Stump Trail dead-ends into the footpath from the right. Continue straight on Brookside Trail to a series of three man-made ponds: Island Pond, Dry Pond, and Big Pond. Trails cross each pond, forming a dam built by local inmates in the 1930s, then they join Brookside Trail. On Big Pond, a dock allows hikers the chance to view waterfowl, amphibians, and reptiles from the lake. There is a large turtle population here, along with geese, ducks, and migratory waterfowl in the spring and fall.

Return to the trail and turn right, walk to the dam, and follow Brookside Trail to the right. There are some good views of the lakeshore to the right as you cross the dam. After the dam, the pathway becomes Back Mountain Trail, and High Springs Trail heads off to the right. Continue on Back Mountain Trail as it begins a moderate-to-difficult climb to a low knob in a piedmont hardwood forest of oak, hickory, sour-wood, sweetgum, black gum, Southern magnolia, and tupelo.

Turn right at the signed intersection at 0.8 miles onto Hickory Stump Trail—a wide, mulch-covered trail—and follow it as it begins to descend the low knob; bear left at the bottom of this easy-to-moderate descent. Turn left onto the marked Crooked Creek Trail at the bottom of the ridge. When Burstin' Heart Trail heads off to the left, Crooked Creek bears right and enters an area of larger trees. The path wraps around a large white oak tree that fell during a storm a couple of years ago. After the oak, the path joins the creek that gives the trail its name. Along the creek's bank, the land has been heavily eroded from recent storms; English ivy abounds here. One upcoming project, according to Weekend Ranger Joe Ledoux, is to replace the nonnative ivy with a native ground cover.

Just past the area of erosion, the path climbs to a wide river plain and splits into two trails, with a third trail (Cypress Spring Trail) heading right at an unmarked intersection. Descend Cypress Spring Trail. After an unmarked trail on the left, which goes to another pond, Cypress Spring Trail splits as it enters a mature-growth forest. Take either footpath—they both lead to a boardwalk that crosses a stream in an area of large trees. As the trail curves right at 1.6 miles, the home of William H. Reynolds comes into view on the right; the barn is straight ahead.

Turn left at the end of the house, then walk around to the front porch. Originally, this was a four-room, two-story home with an enclosed staircase; the judge expanded the home, adding more rooms and an attic. Outbuildings include a barn and sheds, along with farm implements. As the trail leaves the homestead, it becomes paved. Portable comfort stations and picnic tables are near the trail in this area. Turn left at the next intersection and return to the parking area.

■ MORE FUN

A welcome center and the Road to Tara Museum are located in the railroad depot in downtown Jonesboro. The original depot was at the center of the Battle of Jonesboro, a pivotal engagement marking the end of the Atlanta Campaign. The present stone building, built in 1867, replaced the structure destroyed by General Sherman and his army on the March to the Sea in 1864. The depot is open weekdays, 8:30 a.m. to 5:30 p.m., and Saturday, 10 a.m. to 4 p.m. Call (770) 478-4800.

■ TO THE TRAILHEAD

Take I-75 South to Exit 233, Jonesboro Road/GA 54. Turn left at the end of the ramp and travel 0.9 miles to a traffic light. Turn left onto Reynolds Road, and travel 1.1 miles to the nature center's parking lot. There is an overflow parking area at 0.8 miles.

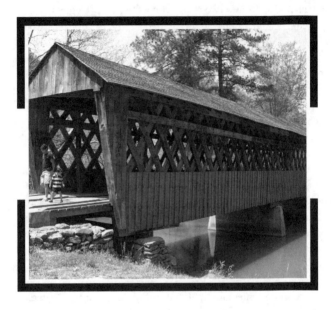

Atlanta North

Chattahoochee Nature Center Trail

■ OVERVIEW

LENGTH: 2.5 miles	noon–5 p.m.; closed Thanksgiving, December 25, and January 1. Admission fee is $5 adults, $4 seniors, $3 children ages 3–12, free for children age 2 and under.
CONFIGURATION: Loop	
SCENERY: Excellent views of Bull Sluice; lake and river views	
EXPOSURE: Full sun in developed areas, mostly shaded elsewhere	**MAPS:** Free with nature center admission fee
TRAFFIC: Moderate	**FACILITIES:** Restrooms, picnic tables
TRAIL SURFACE: Compacted soil, pavement in the developed areas	
HIKING TIME: 1.5 hours	**SPECIAL COMMENTS:** Kids can enjoy Camp Kingfisher during summer weekdays and explore the nature center on instructor-led hikes.
ACCESS: Open year-round, Monday–Saturday, 9 a.m.–5 p.m.; Sunday,	

■ SNAPSHOT

This hike explores the Chattahoochee River above Bull Sluice and then climbs into the watershed. The hike ends at the Discovery Center, where kids can learn about the natural world.

■ CLOSE-UP

Pam and I are frequently asked "Where's a good place to start if I haven't done a lot of hiking?" Chattahoochee Nature Center is our standard answer. Offering a deep-woods experience in an in-town setting, the nature center also has an interpretive center plus natural history and animal exhibits along the trail to keep the kids involved in the hike, with signs identifying many of the trees and plants. We normally hike these trails two or three times a year simply to enjoy the setting. Enter the trail through the Discovery Center and pay the modest admission. As you pass through the attraction, take a look at the ways the

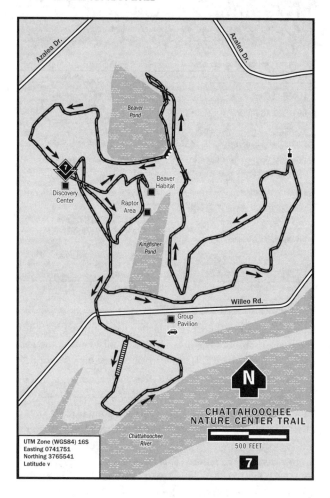

Chattahoochee River runs through our lives and how we can help preserve the river for future generations. Arriving early has an added benefit: large waterfowl can be spotted from a wetlands boardwalk. Follow the asphalt road down to a gated chain-link fence near a traffic light–controlled intersection at 0.2 miles. Cross with the light to a second unlocked chain-link gate on a boardwalk.

Jutting out into the Chattahoochee River, and frequently in full sun, the boardwalk provides ample opportunity to study the unique wetland plant life in the area. Turn right at the first intersection and follow the boardwalk as it wraps around to the left. Bull Sluice Lake on the Chattahoochee River opens up on the right at 0.4 miles, allowing visitors to quietly watch some large waterfowl. On one crisp morning, we spotted a pair of ospreys, a great blue heron, and numerous smaller birds. Named for the waterfall that was completely covered when the lake was formed, Bull Sluice was created by Atlanta's first hydroelectric project, Morgan Falls Dam.

As you continue around the boardwalk loop, head down a short side trail on the right to an A frame–roofed area with seats. Here you can enjoy good long-distance views of the Chattahoochee River before the boardwalk curves around to the left again, where it explores an inland estuary. After returning to the starting point and crossing the road, enter through the chain-link gate and turn right almost immediately, following a concrete path down to an overlook on Kingfisher Pond.

On the left side of the lake is the Discovery Center, where instructor-led sessions allow kids the opportunity to experience various animals and reptiles. As the path continues through "Georgia's Living Wetlands," interpretive displays discuss protecting the fragile environment of the riverine wetlands or riparian zones. Water-loving trees, including river birch, black walnut, and water oak, have been planted to give visitors an idea of what a healthy riverine wetland might look like.

After a second overlook is a re-creation of Southeast Georgia's hardwood and pine forest. Watch for American beech and loblolly pine, which form a canopy over magnolia (Southern grandifolia) and dogwood. A dirt road crosscuts the path where it jogs slightly to the right. A white-blazed crossover trail heads off to the left at 0.9 miles, but continue straight ahead to a Civil War–era grave at 1.1 miles. At the grave, the trail circles to the left, climbing to its highest point, where an orange-blazed trail intersects it. Bear left on the orange trail, which immediately begins to gradually descend.

After passing a white crossover trail on the left, you'll notice an old homestead on the right, made apparent by the home's chimney. After you pass a white crossover trail that heads off to the right, the orange and red trails end. Turn right on the blue-blazed Kingfisher Pond Trail, climbing to an interpretive area at 1.4 miles. A cutaway into the mountain, along with an interpretive sign, displays the layers of soil typical in the piedmont section of Georgia.

Bearing left at a side trail down to an amphitheater, the footpath once again begins an easy climb to a wooden bridge over a gully. Just before the bridge, a white crossover trail joins the footpath from the right, and the bridge makes a 90-degree left-hand turn. As the pathway swings around to the right, an orange-blazed trail joins from the right just before you cross a wooden bridge. Kingfisher Pond Trail ends at Beaver Pond. Bear right on the green-blazed Beaver Pond Trail, which follows the pond's shore as it easily climbs to a bridge at 1.6 miles. After crossing the bridge you'll see houses on the right and the trail quickly ends. Turn around and return to the three-way intersection with the blue trail, but continue on the green trail, turning right and crossing an earthen dam in full sun. On the far side of the dam, a concrete walkway joins the trail on the left, but continue straight to the end of the lake and bear right to the yellow-blazed Stone Cabin Trail at 1.9 miles.

The trail bears left at an open field through a forest that includes sweetgum and tulip poplar and then descends gradually. Turn left and follow the walkway around to the right to reach the Bonnie Baker Butterfly Gardens. Plants in this area have been especially chosen for their ability to attract butterflies. Among the flora are blazing stars, Carolina silverbells, yarrow, purple coneflower, and the aptly named butterfly bush. Briefly returning to the green trail, the concrete walkway then takes a hard right to continue to a side trail on the right that heads down to a beaver habitat. After visiting the beaver, turn around and return to the main trail, where you'll turn left. The pathway leads through a series of raptor aviaries that house injured birds of prey ending at a massive eagle aviary, where a pair of injured American bald eagles spend their time. Follow the trail as it bears right in front of a pavilion.. Follow this road to return to the entrance of the Discovery Center.

■ MORE FUN

Roswell Riverwalk is a lineal park with many access points that follows the Chattahoochee River. It is currently 3 miles in length but is being extended.

■ TO THE TRAILHEAD

Take GA 400 to Exit 6, Northridge Road. Turn west on Northridge and travel 0.4 miles to a right on Roswell Road, which crosses a bridge over the Chattahoochee River at 1.7 miles. At the end of the bridge, turn left on Azalea Drive. Travel 1.9 miles to a traffic light and turn left on Willeo Road. Drive 0.6 miles, then turn right into the Chattahoochee Nature Center and follow the road around to the parking lot.

■ OVERVIEW

LENGTH: 5.6 miles

CONFIGURATION: Out-and-back with a balloon at the end

SCENERY: Civil War battlefield, with the massive Illinois Monument at the site of the heaviest fighting; entrenchments, John Ward Creek

EXPOSURE: Full sun to full shade

TRAFFIC: Moderate

TRAIL SURFACE: Gravel road, compacted dirt, paved road

HIKING TIME: 3 hours

ACCESS: Open year-round; hours vary depending on season

MAPS: Available in Kennesaw Mountain Visitors Center; USGS Marietta

FACILITIES: None

SPECIAL COMMENTS: There are a number of interpretive markers throughout the hike with extensive information on the battle of Kennesaw Mountain. The paved-road portion of the hike has both markers and monuments and runs just east of the actual battle line in the area.

■ SNAPSHOT

The trail follows a gravel road from Burnt Hickory Road to Dallas Highway, then parallels a low ridge to Cheatham Hill. After taking you to explore Civil War entrenchments, the trail descends to Kolb's Farm Trail, returning to Dallas Highway along a paved road. On the return to the trailhead, the hike leaves the main trunk and explores the watershed of Noses Creek.

■ CLOSE-UP

General Sherman's Atlanta Campaign in the Civil War had stalled at the western side of Kennesaw Mountain. To the south, Confederate General John Bell Hood had prevented Sherman's favorite move, an end run around the Confederate line at Kolb's Farm. Now the massive army was sitting beneath the bastion of Kennesaw Mountain. Feeding the army was a logistical nightmare: Deep in enemy territory, some of Sher-

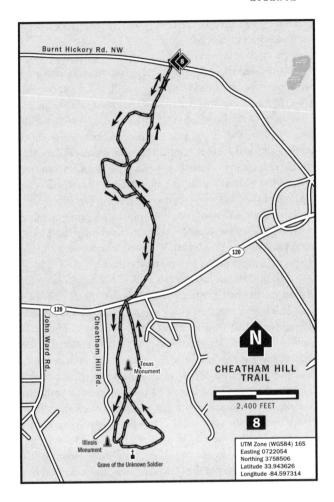

man's men were up to 8 miles from the railhead. Sherman decided to launch an assault against a broad front stretching from the base of Big Kennesaw down to Cheatham Hill. He hoped to find a hole in the Confederate line—an improbable situation, given that his adversary was General Joseph Johnston, an expert at defense.

As dawn broke on June 27, 1864, the Union Army began the coordinated attack against Rebel entrenchments, starting at Big Kennesaw and quickly moving south to Cheatham Hill. The trail roughly follows just west of the main Confederate line from south of Pigeon Hill to Cheatham Hill. At the start of the hike, a field on the left just past a split-rail fence is where Union soldiers attacked a Rebel skirmish line manned by the recently transferred Georgia 63rd Regiment. The skirmish line was designed to warn troops of the approaching enemy. However, the men of the 63rd stood their ground against an overwhelming force. As the Confederate line evaporated, other members of the regiment charged, only adding to the carnage. Still, as the Union line neared the Rebels, it slowed, eventually withdrawing because the position became unsustainable.

On the left, an interpretive marker has additional information on the battle. After passing the first field, Cheatham Hill Trail begins climbing along a gravel road, with alternating cleared fields that tend to attract a wide variety of birds. The trail descends, quickly entering a pine forest (mostly shortleaf and loblolly) with white oak and American beech, a typical second-growth forest of the Georgia piedmont. At the start of the hike, there are some large post oaks; hickory joins the mix later on. At the bottom of the first hill, the road crosses a stone bridge then climbs as it curves, first to the right then back to the left. At 0.3 miles the return footpath heads off to the right, promptly followed by another side trail on the left after the last field. From this point to the Dallas Highway, the wide road runs through the forest but is only occasionally shaded.

At Noses Creek (named for Chief Noses, a Cherokee who lived near the creek), the roadway crosses the clear stream on a wooden bridge with no rail. Notice the stonework supports under the bridge, which obviously predate the current structure. Following along the creek, the gravel road begins an extended moderate climb in full sun to Dallas Highway. Be careful crossing Dallas Highway—the intersection has no traffic light, and people tend to speed through the Kennesaw Mountain area.

After crossing Dallas Highway, the trail passes through a split-rail fence, and immediately on the right is a sign indicating that Cheatham Hill and Kolb's Farm are straight ahead. After a short stretch through a mostly pine forest, the trail breaks out into the full sun of an open field, 50 to 100 feet west of the paved-road entrance to Cheatham Hill. On the morning of June 27, 1864, there was fighting along a line between where the path and the road now run.

Entering an area of a fairly extensive pine blowdown at 1.8 miles, the trail dips to adjoin the paved road at an artillery battery at 2 miles, separated from the traffic by a brown gate to prevent vehicular access. Off to the left is the Cheatham Hill parking lot, but the path continues straight ahead, and you soon reach an open field. At a four-way intersection in the middle of the field, turn left and climb to the Illinois Monument, a large, bold memorial to the men under the command of Union General George Thomas who were ordered to charge Cheatham Hill. After climbing the steps and viewing the monument, circle around to the left. There is an improved tunnel below the monument, dug by Union soldiers who were going to try to blow a hole in the Confederate line.

As you circle to the left of the monument, the path climbs to a series of Confederate entrenchments known as the Dead Angle. Hundred of bodies of Union soldiers who charged the Rebels were strewn in front of the entrenchments, but the Confederate line held, handing the Union Army its worst defeat of the Atlanta Campaign. At the top of the hill, turn left and follow the path along the entrenchments until you come to Mebane's battery, an artillery position that anchored the right end of Benjamin Franklin Cheatham's line. The hill was named in his honor following the success of the Confederate army.

Turn around, keeping the Illinois Monument on your right as you follow the footpath curving to the left along the ridge. At the end of the ridge, the trail begins an extended moderate descent, passing the grave of an unknown soldier who was discovered by Civilian Conservation Corps (CCC) workers who were improving the area in the 1930s. At 2.8 miles Cheatham Hill Trail turns left, joining Kolb's Farm Loop for 0.1 mile as it continues to descend. At the second intersection, Kolb's Farm Trail turns right, and Cheatham Hill goes straight, quickly curving left and beginning a moderate climb to a parking lot at 3.1 miles. From here, follow the paved road that bears right and walk past a series of interpretive markers and monuments before crossing Dallas Highway.

After crossing the bridge over Noses Creek, turn left on a compacted-dirt path that enters the full shade of a diverse hardwood forest that runs between the creek on the left and a forested wetlands on the right. At 4.6 miles the trail turns right and begins to climb into the watershed of Noses Creek on a good thigh-burner to the top of a knoll. From here the trail begins a series of easy up-and-downs; turn left on the main trunk at 5.3 miles to return to the trailhead.

■ TO THE TRAILHEAD

Take I-75 North to Exit 263, GA 120/Marietta/Roswell, known locally as the South 120 Loop. Two exits head off the two-lane exit road before it rejoins I-75. You want the second exit, labeled Marietta/Southern Poly, which heads off to the right after the overpass. The road curves sharply around to the right before joining GA 120. At 2.8 miles turn right on South Marietta Parkway, which is also the 120 Loop. Drive 0.2 miles and turn left on Whitlock Avenue (GA 120). Turn left on Burnt Hickory Road at the Coldwell Banker office and Whitlock Package Store, at 1.2 miles. At 1.1 miles the road enters the Kennesaw Mountain National Battlefield Park; go 0.4 miles; there is parallel parking on the left.

■ OVERVIEW

LENGTH: 3.5 miles	**HIKING TIME:** 2.5 hours
CONFIGURATION: Out-and-back	**ACCESS:** Open year-round
SCENERY: This trail features great riverside views most of the way, rising near the end to afford an excellent "above-it-all" view. There are historic buildings near the trail.	**MAPS:** USGS Mableton
	FACILITIES: Restrooms are available at the visitor center at the start of the hike; there are picnic tables along the hike.
EXPOSURE: Shaded, except for initial 0.3 miles, which is in full sun	**SPECIAL COMMENTS:** This area developed into an industrial center because of water power and the nearby Western and Atlantic Railroad.
TRAFFIC: Moderate	
TRAIL SURFACE: Gravel road turning to packed dirt at the end	

■ SNAPSHOT

This historic road explores a portion of Confederate general Joseph Johnston's Smyrna Line and the remains of an old woolen mill. Hikers can view Ruff's Mill and continue on to see Concord Covered Bridge.

■ CLOSE-UP

From the parking lot, walk toward the stone and wood interpretive center. Here there is detailed information on the historic sites along the trail in addition to a viewing platform that overlooks the wetland marsh formed by Nickajack Creek. From the building, walk to the northwest corner of the parking area, where the trail enters the woods and gradually descends a compacted-soil trail. After an S-curve at the start of the treadway, two immense beech trees on either side of the path shade the area. A small overlook allows you to inspect the lower beech tree.

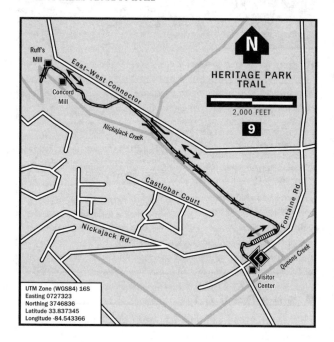

Next, the path gradually declines to a marsh that is traversed by a wooden boardwalk. It's easy to spot various smaller wetland birds here. About 200 feet farther along, a more substantial iron bridge with wooden planking carries you across Nickajack Creek. Look to the left as you cross and you'll see water cascading over shoals. Immediately after the end of the bridge, turn left at an unmarked intersection of four trails.

Now a gravel road, the trail begins to parallel Nickajack Creek on the left. Following the battle of Kennesaw Mountain, Confederate General Joseph Johnston pulled back to a secondary defensive position known as the Smyrna Line. Nickajack Creek formed the southern end of the line. Soldiers stationed on this part of the trail on July 3, 1864, came under artillery fire in the morning. This was the only fighting in this vicinity.

First in a series of scenic creekside shots comes into view at 0.4 miles. Photographers will want to get here before noon for the best pictures. Shortly past the scenic view, houses are visible across the creek and up a hill. At 0.5 miles the trail crosses the first of a string of small wooden bridges across tributaries of Nickajack Creek. Immediately after the first bridge, there is a side trail to the right. The bridge at 1.1 miles is longer than the others, spanning a creek, a wetland area, and another creek. On an early-fall morning, it is possible to see a number of large waterfowl in this area.

About 0.2 miles after the wetlands, the pathway makes an abrupt left turn, and the traffic noise grows very loud. At this point, the East–West Connector, a major Cobb County thoroughfare, is up the embankment to the right. A few steps past the turn is a picnic table, and just beyond the table is an excellent view of the creek. The far riverbank is a wall of river-worn granite, common in the Georgia piedmont. As you continue down the treadway, the traffic noise subsides. At 1.6 miles the historic woolen mill comes into view.

The water from Nickajack Creek powered Concord Woolen Mills, a three-story building made of fieldstone and cement. Today only a portion of the mill remains. Built before the Civil War by Robert Daniel and Martin Ruff, the mill produced wool for the Confederacy and was among Sherman's targets during the Atlanta Campaign. Union soldiers destroyed it in 1864 shortly after they captured it. Following the war, the mill incorporated and was rebuilt. In 1872 the western Georgia industrialist Seaborn Love and others purchased the mill and a portion of the surrounding land that included housing for mill workers.

In 1910 Annie (Gillespie) Johnson tried to bring in Russian Jews who were part of the Galveston movement to revitalize the mill. Unfortunately, her request for help was rejected; the mill was abandoned and fell into disrepair. When the East–West Connector and the nearby Silver Comet Trail were built, metal supports were added to what remained of the building to ensure that blasting would not further damage the walls. Take time to explore the woolen mill and an adjacent outbuilding.

Returning to the path, you'll find two unmarked paved trails heading off to the right as you pass the mill. These connect Heritage Park to Silver Comet Trail, a mixed-use paved trail. As you continue, the path begins to slowly and steadily rise; there are a number of side trails to both the left and the right. At 1.7 miles there is a long-distance view from the trail, which is now 100 feet above Nickajack Creek. Five hundred feet farther on, the trail makes a hard left turn and begins an easy descent to Ruff's Mill and Concord Bridge.

Known as Daniel and Ruff Mill when it was built before the Civil War, by the time Sherman's troops arrived in 1864 the mill was known simply as Ruff's Mill. Unlike the woolen mill, Ruff's gristmill survived the Union invasion and prospered after the war, eventually being sold and run as Martin's Feed and Grain. When Asbury Martin left, he moved lock, stock, and millworks to another site, so all that is left is the mill building, along with the miller's house, both of which are privately owned.

At the roadway, turn left and walk down about 100 feet to the Concord Covered Bridge. One of the shorter remaining covered bridges in Georgia, Concord spans 130 feet between two stone abutments. Two modern concrete piers give the heavily used covered bridge additional support in the center. This 1872 bridge features queen-post trusses and was completely renovated in 1983.

An earlier structure spanned Nickajack Creek in this spot as early as 1848. On July 3, 1864, Confederate soldiers stationed on high ground just south of the bridge came under Union attack. They were driven from the ridge, crossed Concord Bridge, and reformed a line on the north side of Nickajack Creek. The following day, the battle of Ruff's Mill was fought about a mile and a half from the mill.

This is the end of the hike. Turn around and retrace your steps to the car.

■ MORE FUN

The Silver Comet Trail that connects to Heritage Park at Concord Woolen Mill is a paved, multiuse trail open every day from dawn to dusk.

■ TO THE TRAILHEAD

Take I-20 West to Exit 51B (I-285 North). Travel north to South Cobb Drive (Exit 15). At the end of the ramp, turn left and drive 1.3 miles to the East–West Connector. Turn left and get in the left-hand lane. Fontaine Road heads off to the left at 2.5 miles. After turning left, travel 0.4 miles to the entrance to Heritage Park on the right. Follow the parking lot around to the far side of the visitor center.

10 *Homestead Trail*

■ OVERVIEW

LENGTH: 5.7 miles	**ACCESS:** Daily, 7 a.m.–10 p.m.
CONFIGURATION: Balloon	**MAPS:** Handout available at trailhead and in visitor center
SCENERY: Multiple views of Lake Allatoona and its tributaries	**FACILITIES:** Restrooms at trailhead
EXPOSURE: Mostly shaded	**SPECIAL COMMENTS:** Red Top Mountain is a popular stop in the Georgia State Park system, with a lodge and restaurant, multiple hiking trails, a marina, and a beach.
TRAFFIC: Moderate	
TRAIL SURFACE: Mulched, compacted soil with few rocks or roots	
HIKING TIME: 3 hours	

■ SNAPSHOT

This hike explores a peninsula of Lake Allatoona and the lake's watershed.

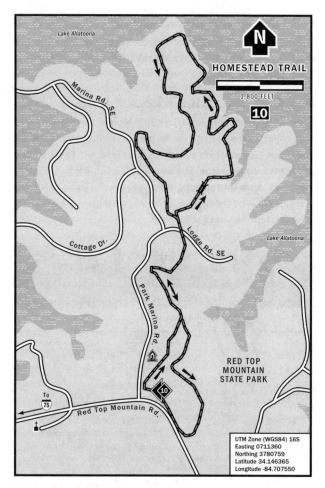

Lake Allatoona

N

HOMESTEAD TRAIL

1,800 FEET

10

Marina Rd. SE

Lodge Rd. SE

Lake Allatoona

Cottage Dr.

Park Marina Rd.

RED TOP
MOUNTAIN
STATE PARK

To
75

Red Top Mountain Rd.

10

UTM Zone (WGS84) 16S
Easting 0711360
Northing 3780759
Latitude 34.146365
Longitude -84.707550

■ CLOSE-UP

Red Top Mountain State Park lies on a peninsula that was slated
to be part of I-75, but local residents strongly objected to the
destruction of this beautiful area, so the state and federal governments rerouted I-75 to the west and preserved the state

park. The name Red Top comes from the presence of iron in the Georgia clay. Today, in addition to 12 miles of hiking trails, the 1,562-acre park contains a lodge and conference center, camping and RV sites, a beach (in season), a boating dock, picnic areas, and group shelters.

Homestead Trail begins in front of the visitor center, heading off on the left as you approach the building. A few steps down the path, you'll find a trailhead kiosk with information about the park and some of the animals you may see on your journey. The path soon passes a ranger residence and a side trail to a group shelter, both on the left side of the path as it continues to drop into a valley through a fair few trees with southern pine beetle damage.

Just short of 0.4 miles, Sweet Gum Trail heads off to the right at a marked intersection. Between the visitor center and the road to the lodge, Sweet Gum Trail and Homestead Trail run parallel. Normally separated by a valley, they share the path for 200 feet here. Sweet Gum Trail bears right at a sign that says simply "Lodge."

Once Sweet Gum Trail leaves, Homestead Trail makes a U-turn, rises at an easy-to-moderate grade, and then makes a second U-turn. As the treadway follows the curve of the hill around to the left, you'll begin to notice orange blazes and interpretive signs. Just past a boardwalk over a wet area, the footpath makes an easy climb to and across Lodge Road. Just after the road, a second lodge trail heads off to the right as Homestead Trail descends to the start of the loop.

The loop can be hiked in either direction, but we chose to walk it counterclockwise because a small hiker sign had an arrow pointing that way. Skirting a valley on the right, the treadway passes the lodge's wastewater-treatment plant, which is on the right-hand side of the path. Watch for an area of impressive sweetgum trees near the plant. The sweetgum tree was important to the Cherokee who inhabited the area before the settlers moved in. They chewed the hardened resin of the tree, and boiled its fruits and leaves to make a medicinal tea. They also mixed the tree's gum with beef tallow to create a salve for wounds.

A tributary of the Etowah River forms on the right as the trail gradually descends. The valley begins to widen and the number of rock outcroppings increases, but the trail curves left and heads away from the creek. As the path turns right, it crosses a bridge, then returns to the tributary, which now has taken on the appearance of a dry lake bottom. When Lake Allatoona is full, this should be a shallow arm. As you continue around the side of the mountain to the left, Lake Allatoona comes into full view at 1.4 miles.

Proposed in the 1930s, the construction of Lake Allatoona began in 1941, only to be delayed by World War II. Built as a watershed lake, Allatoona was designed to hold back the waters of the Etowah River that had regularly flooded the city of Rome, Georgia. During the fall and winter, when rainfall is at its lowest, the lake is partially drained. Spring rains fill the lake instead of inundating the relatively flat land of the Etowah River Valley. In 1947, only months before the dam was complete, the Etowah flooded for the last time.

Coming out on the first peninsula at 1.6 miles, Homestead Trail gently curves left. Returning to a cove, the pathway crosses a rivulet on a wooden bridge and then returns down another finger of the lake. This pattern will be repeated throughout the lake portion of the hike. About halfway through the second peninsula, there are a number of rock outcroppings, and the number and size of nearby boulders increase. A few feet past the 2-mile marker a trail on the right descends a moderate slope to the lakeshore. After passing this side trail, the main trail turns in to a cove, makes another U-turn, and returns to the lake. Now making an extended run alongside but above the lake, the trail gently curves left and begins to climb away from the lake. At 2.7 miles a blue-blazed trail heads off Homestead Trail on the right, running toward the lake. This is the final access point to the lake on the pathway.

Running inland, the trail makes easy-to-moderate up-and-down climbs, normally ascending 50 feet or so before falling by about the same amount. As the trail climbs to 3.5 miles, a blue-blazed trail heads off to the left. Take just a few more steps, and Homestead Trail curves right and begins to descend into a valley. The treadway also becomes somewhat rocky for the first time. As it begins climbing, Homestead Trail winds to the left, rising and straightening as it nears the top of the mountain. Look down on the left, and you will see the trail you walked earlier. From this point, it's an easy walk to the start of the loop. Turn right and continue down the trail to the second intersection with Sweet Gum Trail, at 4.9 miles. Homestead Trail curves to the right as Sweet Gum Trail goes straight before bearing left, then paralleling Homestead Trail on the other side of a valley. At 5.2 miles Sweet Gum Trail reaches a four-way intersection. Turn left onto the visitor center loop. This easy return trail is a slightly longer return route to the Red Top Mountain visitor center parking lot. After it curves around to an overlook, the trail continues a moderate climb through a boulder field to Red Top Mountain Road. Turn right and return to the trailhead parking lot.

■ MORE FUN

Cartersville is home to the world-class Booth Western Art Museum. One of the finest collections of Western and Civil War art, the Booth Museum also has an exhibit on the presidents of the United States that features a brief biography, a photograph or painting, and a signed sample of each man's handwriting. Take I-75 North to Exit 288, Main Street. Turn left and travel 2.3 miles. Turn left at Wall Street and follow the signs for two blocks to the parking area.

■ TO THE TRAILHEAD

Take I-75 North to Exit 285, Red Top Mountain Road. At the end of the ramp, turn right and travel 1.8 miles to the visitor center.

■ OVERVIEW

LENGTH: 2.9 miles	**ACCESS:** Open year-round
CONFIGURATION: Double loop	**MAPS:** There is a map at the kiosk at the trailhead, USGS Buford Dam
SCENERY: Some winter views of the Chattahoochee River	**FACILITIES:** Restrooms and picnicking nearby
EXPOSURE: Full sun at start, then mostly shaded	**SPECIAL COMMENTS:** Dogs are not allowed to cross into the Bowman
TRAFFIC: Low	Island Unit of the Chattahoochee River National Recreation Area, nor are they
TRAIL SURFACE: Mostly gravel roads connected by compacted dirt	allowed in Buford Dam Park. This hike never crosses on to Bowman's Island.
HIKING TIME: 1.5 hours	

■ SNAPSHOT

This double-loop trail in the Bowman Island Unit of the Chattahoochee River National Recreation Area circles just below the crest of two hills south of the Buford Dam. Horseback riding is allowed, but this section of the trail is only lightly used.

■ CLOSE-UP

At the south end of the first parking lot, a modular bridge has been placed over Haw Creek (or McClain's Branch). After crossing the creek, the pathway bears right, crossing a wide, level field that was once a part of the Chattahoochee River floodplain. At 0.1 mile a second path heads off to the right, almost doubling back on the trail as it begins an easy-to-moderate climb to an old road that circles the top of a low hill. Once on this road, there is some elevation change as the pathway climbs and falls, in and out of coves. Much of the pine cover has fallen prey to the pine borer, but there are still some good stands of longleaf. You can see a few homes behind trees, but for the most part they are not obtrusive.

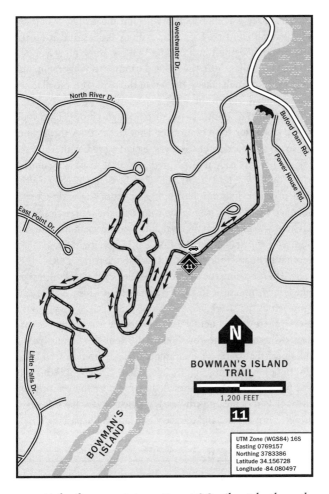

At the three-way intersection at 0.8 miles, take the pathway that bears left and climbs to the top of the ridge. From
here the path drops rapidly but not steeply, finally curving
hard to the right and dropping to a wide road 0.3 miles later.
Continue straight, following the gravel road as it climbs to

another three-way intersection 0.1 mile ahead. The trail turns left, leaving the first loop and joining the second loop 0.3 miles later. Turn left and cross a shallow creek on a wooden bridge 1.5 miles into the hike. Dammed downstream, the river forms a small lake to the left of the path. You can also see homes ahead and on the right.

As the trail follows an old road through a mostly hardwood forest, watch for the occasionally large beech trees throughout the hike. The barrage of oak trees, including red, white, and pin oak, and an occasional maple tree, is typical of a Georgia piedmont forest. The trail drops, and off to the right you can hear the rush of water. In some places you can spot the wide Chattahoochee River, especially in the winter. As the trail circles to the left, it moves away from the river and climbs back to the intersection with the trail from the first loop. Turn right, then make another right and follow the road back to the parking lot.

After crossing the bridge at the start of the trail, turn right and follow the creek to the Chattahoochee River. As the trail turns left at the riverbank, you can usually see the shoals in the center; there are frequently waterfowl on or near them, even if a trout fisherman is nearby. Follow the trail to the left, past a "blooper" that warns of an imminent release from Buford Dam. Continue on, moving slightly inland and crossing a boat ramp and picnic area to a prefabricated bridge over the powerhouse channel. Part of the powerhouse is visible from the left side of the bridge. Turn around and retrace your steps to the parking lot.

■ MORE FUN

The visitor center at the Buford Dam Office provides information on the creation of the dam, facts about Lake Lanier, and a general history of the area around the lake. It is open daily, 8 a.m. to 4:30 p.m. Call (770) 945-9531 for more information.

■ TO THE TRAILHEAD

Take GA 400 North to Exit 14, Buford/Cumming. The exit ramp passes under the overpass, then loops around. Turn right and travel 0.3 miles to GA 9. Turn right (at Burger King and Wachovia) and travel 0.9 miles to Buford Dam Road. Turn right at the Shell station. Drive 4.8 miles, until Buford Dam Road makes a 90-degree left-hand turn; you'll see a wide drive-way straight ahead. As you enter the apron, a sign for Lower Pool Park is almost straight ahead. Continue on this dirt road 0.2 miles to the first parking lot on the right. The trailhead is on the north end of the lot.

12   Jones Bridge Trail

■ OVERVIEW

LENGTH: 5.2 miles

CONFIGURATION: Loop

SCENERY: Historic bridge, riverside views

EXPOSURE: Full sun in the vicinity of the historic bridge, full shade else-where

TRAFFIC: Heavy near the bridge; mod-erate down to the boat launch; light south of the launch

TRAIL SURFACE: Compacted soil

HIKING TIME: 2 hours

ACCESS: Open year-round, dawn–dusk

MAPS: Available at park headquarters at Island Ford; USGS Norcross, Duluth, Chamblee

FACILITIES: Restrooms, boat launch, some picnic tables, fishing dock

SPECIAL COMMENTS: Jones Bridge was a privately owned toll bridge that was built in 1904 and ceased opera-tion in 1922. Before that time, a ferry crossed the river at roughly the same spot.

■ SNAPSHOT

This hike explores Jones Bridge and climbs into nearby hills that allow long-distance views of some of Atlanta's most expen-

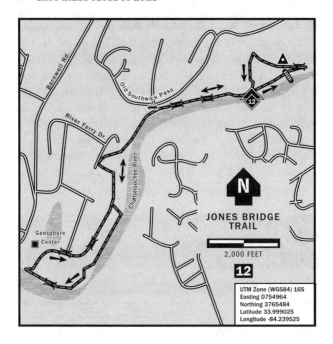

sive homes and then follows the floodplain of the Chatta-hoochee, climbing to explore a ridge and returning to loop around a second floodplain.

■ CLOSE-UP

Ferries were the first privately owned businesses to span Geor-gia's mighty rivers. With increased competition from railroads, ferry owners began to build bridges and charge a toll for cross-ing. As the government began building roads in the 1920s, many of the old bridges quickly became obsolete. Jones Bridge's usefulness (in the mind of its owner) came to an end in the early 1920s, when it was abandoned, although farmers did con-tinue to use it until the wooden planking rotted. In 1940 World

War II sent scrap metal prices soaring, even though the United States had not entered the war yet. A group of workmen began dismantling the southern end of Jones Bridge, working in plain sight one day. People didn't ask any questions until the men didn't show up the second day. Then folks realized that the workers had made off with the scrap metal, and probably sold it a piece at a time so that their theft would go undetected in the lucrative Atlanta market.

From the trailhead kiosk, follow a wide dirt road to make an easy descent through a diverse hardwood forest to a four-way intersection 200 feet from the start. Take a minute to walk down to the riverbank, straight ahead, and enjoy the view of the Chattahoochee. On returning, turn right and follow the riverbank, keeping the river on your right. The trail runs some 20 feet inside the bank, and large rock outcroppings tell the river's story. As you pass the outcroppings on the left, take a close look at the water-worn edges and eroded strata in the rock. Before the river was controlled by Buford Dam—20 miles north as the river flows—water levels would fluctuate much more than they do today. The rock, which would be covered only in an unusual circumstance today, routinely flooded before 1953. As you continue along the trail, the floodplain opens up into a park, and a dock for both fishing and viewing extends into the river, on your right. In the distance the half-span of Jones Bridge waits for another crew to finish the job begun in 1940.

Continue straight ahead toward the bridge past a trail on the left and over a wooden bridge that crosses a stream. Finally, as you approach an intrusive chain-link fence, you'll reach the bridge, which juts out over the Chattahoochee River. Jones Bridge Road, which is still a major road in north Fulton County, ran to this point, crossed the river on the bridge, and continued on the south side of the Chattahoochee. There are a number of large pines in the area. The trail continues a short way along the riverbank, next to the fence.

From the bridge turn around and begin walking the inside of the open field toward a creek crossing and map stand. After the wet-foot crossing, the path joins a road that bears right and begins to climb into the forest. As the trail begins a moderate ascent, it curves away from the riverbank. At 0.8 miles the climb eases as the roadway runs nearly level at the ridgetop. An easy descent returns you to the north end of the parking lot. Continue to the trailhead, but turn right and follow the riverbank, keeping the Chattahoochee on the left. Here the floodplain is wider, not constrained by the hills adjacent to the river. We flushed a blue heron at the first bridge, just after the turn.

Crossing another wooden bridge at 1.3 miles, the pathway takes you to a third bridge and the fishing-ramp parking area 0.3 miles later. Walk straight across the lot, and the path continues, almost immediately crossing another bridge. Turning inland at 1.8 miles at a flight of wooden steps, the trail begins another moderate climb into the Chattahoochee River watershed, dropping to a gravel road, and then climbing again. Notice the American beech trees at the top of the mountain some 0.2 miles after the start of the climb. There are four or five massive beech trees, and much smaller ones in the nearby forest. As the pathway begins to descend, you'll see a home on the left, between the trail and the river.

Come to a three-way intersection with a map stand at 2.3 miles, turn left, and continue an easy descent toward the river, coming to a second intersection a couple hundred feet later. Take the trail on the right, which runs fairly level down to a wooden bridge at 2.6 miles. The footpath curves gently right, and a crossover trail heads off to the left. Just past the crossover trail is an intersection, where the trail bears left; next, you come to a bridge as you enter an open field near the Geosphere Center. At a grassy road leading to the center, turn left; the trail begins an easy descent, curving right at a map stand at 3 miles, then making a hard left less than 0.1 mile later.

After following the riverbank another 0.1 mile, the foot-path curves left, away from the bank, to a right-hand turn at a three-way intersection, crossing a bridge, making another right and then yet another right-hand turn as the trail rejoins the river at 3.2 miles. After passing two side trails on the left, take a few steps up to a low ridge in an area of large trees. As the trail bears left, a trail heads off to the right, then the foot-path curves right and another trail comes in from the right. At 3.9 miles the pathway crosscuts a historic road; look for a map stand 100 feet to the left, and follow the trail to it. Turn right and retrace your steps to the car.

■ TO THE TRAILHEAD

Take GA 400 North to Holcomb Bridge Road/140 East. Turn right at the end of the ramp. Travel 4.2 miles to Barnwell Road (there's a CVS and a SunTrust Bank on the corner). Ignore the first brown sign, which is the entrance to the Environmental Center. At 1.6 miles turn right at the Jones Bridge Unit sign. Fol-low the road as it curves around and switches back, passing a small parking lot on the right for cars with fishing boats. At 1.2 miles the main parking lot opens up. Turn left, park, and return to the trailhead kiosk on the south end of the parking lot.

■ OVERVIEW

LENGTH: 2.3 miles	**HIKING TIME:** 1 hour; Heritage Farm tour adds 1 hour
CONFIGURATION: Loop	
SCENERY: Meadowlands, Heritage Farm	**ACCESS:** Open year-round, dawn–dusk
	MAPS: Available at trailhead and in interpreted farm area; USGS Norcross/Luxomni
EXPOSURE: Full sun	
TRAFFIC: Moderate	**FACILITIES:** Restrooms at trailhead
TRAIL SURFACE: Paved with asphalt, except in the Heritage Farm	**SPECIAL COMMENTS:** In spring the meadow is full of color.

■ SNAPSHOT

McDaniel Farm Park is built around a subsistence farm similar to many of the farms in the area. In addition to the asphalt trail and a free self-guided tour of the farm, there is a heritage tour that is interpreted by docents on Tuesday, Thursday, and Saturday that takes in the farmhouse.

■ CLOSE-UP

When people think of antebellum Georgia, most picture the massive coastal cotton plantations. In the Atlanta area, however, most agriculture before the Civil War was subsistence farming, raising enough corn and wheat to meet only the family's needs. The grain products from these farms had to be cracked or ground before being consumed; wealthier planters coined the derogatory term "cracker" to describe the poorer farmers. Atlantans, though, were proud of the term: For more than 60 years, "Cracker" was the name of its minor league baseball team. Although the McDaniel family owned the farm from 1859 until it was given to the county after Archie McDaniel's death in 1999,

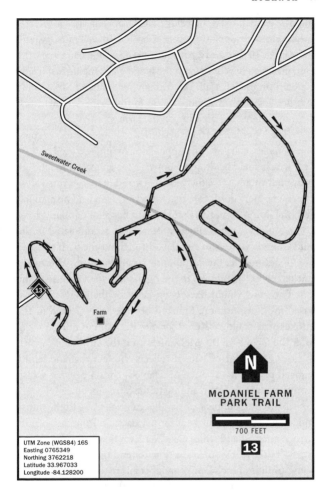

McDANIEL FARM
PARK TRAIL

700 FEET

13

UTM Zone (WGS84) 16S
Easting 0765349
Northing 3762218
Latitude 33.967033
Longitude -84.128200

the farm is set up as a 1930s farm might have been.

From the kiosk adjacent to the facilities, head left, following the asphalt path as it curves 180 degrees, passing a group shelter on the left before crossing a wooden bridge over a deep ravine. Watch for some larger trees here, including tulip poplar and oak. As you cross the bridge, the farm's entrance is directly ahead. Guided tours are given every Tuesday, Thursday, and Saturday at 10 a.m. and 2 p.m. and cost $3. If you can't make the tour, pick up a brochure from the metal pail hanging just inside the barn on the left wall. We strongly recommend the walking tour because it gives visitors access to the farmhouse, which is the most interesting building on the farm.

The lower level of the barn is used to house animals—cows, horses, mules, and pigs. The upper floor, or loft, was used to store feed, which could be dropped down to the animals through specially built chutes. On either side are two additional covered areas where a farmer could store machinery or extra feed he couldn't fit in the loft. Also notice that the barn has a lot of open spaces in the building; these allowed the air that accumulated in the mild Georgia winters to circulate throughout the barn all year.

Continue to the farmhouse straight ahead. There is a chicken coop (henhouse) to the right and a smokehouse to the left. The hens would have been kept for their eggs and not raised for consumption. Smoked or salted meat cured in the smokehouse could be stored for months without refrigeration. After the Civil War, the McDaniels built the farmhouse, which is directly in front of you; it reflects the fact that the family enjoyed prosperity. For the McDaniels, cotton became a cash crop after the Civil War, adding to the farm's income.

Notice an old pear tree and pecan tree close to the house and a Chinese chestnut a bit farther back. In front and on the far side are post and white oak. The lawn is swept—there is no grass—because it would take time to tend the lawn. Inside the home, photos of each family member adorn the rooms in which they slept, and letters written home by the boys during World War II are simply addressed "McDaniel, Duluth, Georgia."

Circle the farmhouse and return to the barn. Once through the barn, turn right on the asphalt path. Known as Cross Park Trail, the path begins a moderate descent to Sweetwater Creek, passing a trail to the parking lot on the right at 0.4

miles. At the bottom of the hill, just before the bridge over the creek, the return trail from the loop enters from the right.

This portion of the path was once a county roadway, but almost all evidence of this fact has been obliterated. Only in the vicinity of the farmhouse is the road evident. From the bridge the path begins to climb, bearing left at 0.7 miles at a three-way intersection. The path continues to a maintenance area, where it turns right to become Wildflower Trail. From a ridge just under a mile into the hike, you can see commercial development off to the left. At this point the trail begins an easy descent as it curves left toward a forested area with a variety of large pines.

After the trees, meadowland, where the McDaniels once planted cotton fields, has been planted to provide color in the spring. Cotton was grown on the farm only until the 1920s, when the boll weevil infestation reached Gwinnett County. After about 1925 the McDaniels planted corn, okra, and butter beans in these fields.

When a path heads off to the right at 1.4 miles, continue straight to another pedestrian bridge over Sweetwater Creek, less than 0.1 mile ahead. After the bridge the trail wraps around to the right and returns to Cross Park Trail. Turn left and climb the hill to an alternate return trail to the parking lot at 2 miles. Turn left on the level path as it swings around McDaniel Farm's outer perimeter. The small house on the right at 2.2 miles was used by the tenant farmer who worked on McDaniel Farm in exchange for food and a small amount of money ($5 for all the work he did for a winter in the 1930s, according to a display inside the house). Notice the outhouse adjacent to the tenant's house. Continue on the trail to the parking lot.

■ MORE FUN

Turn left onto old Norcross Road, then turn left at the first traffic light. Gwinnett Place Mall is on your right. Gwinnett Place features major anchor stores like Sears and Macy's and many smaller upscale shops. For rail fans, return to Pleasant Hill Road and turn right, then turn right at Buford Highway for the South-eastern Railway Museum.

■ TO THE TRAILHEAD

Take I-85 North to Exit 103, Steve Reynolds Boulevard. Turn left at the end of the ramp and travel 1.1 miles, then turn right at Atlanta Toyota onto Old Norcross Road. At 0.6 miles turn left onto McDaniel Farm Road, just before the Land Rover dealership. Be careful—it's a divided highway that is not clearly marked. In 0.3 miles the road curves to the left and enters the parking lot for McDaniel Farm Park.

 14 Stone Mountain Loop

■ OVERVIEW

LENGTH: 5.5 miles

CONFIGURATION: Loop

SCENERY: Multiple views of Stone Mountain and the Confederate Memorial, the world's largest carving; a gristmill, covered bridge, streams, and lakeshore

EXPOSURE: Full sun in the area of the memorial and in multiple areas where the trail runs on granite, mostly shaded elsewhere

TRAFFIC: Heavy between Confederate Hall and Sky Lift, light elsewhere

TRAIL SURFACE: Compacted soil, Chattahoochee stone, granite

HIKING TIME: 2.5 hours

ACCESS: Open year-round

MAPS: Request the hiking map when purchasing your parking pass ($7); an additional map is available at Confederate Hall; USGS Stone Mountain

FACILITIES: Restrooms at the trailhead and at most attractions; playgrounds, picnic tables

SPECIAL COMMENTS: Scouts can earn merit badges for hiking this trail. Stop by Confederate Hall for details. While inside the park, be sure to visit the Antebellum Plantation and the Carillon Bells, the only major attractions not on the Stone Mountain Loop. Phone (770) 498-5690.

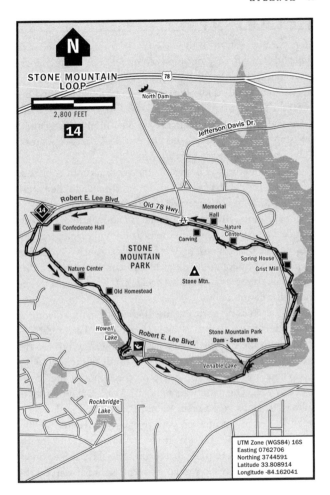

N

STONE MOUNTAIN LOOP

2,800 FEET

14

North Dam

78

Jefferson Davis Dr.

Robert E. Lee Blvd.

Old 78 Hwy.

Memorial Hall

14

Confederate Hall

Nature Center

Carving

STONE MOUNTAIN PARK

Nature Center

Old Homestead

Stone Mtn.

Spring House

Grist Mill

Howell Lake

Robert E. Lee Blvd.

Stone Mountain Park Dam - South Dam

Venable Lake

Rockbridge Lake

UTM Zone (WGS84) 16S
Easting 0762706
Northing 3744591
Latitude 33.808914
Longitude -84.162041

■ SNAPSHOT

This loop trail takes visitors to most of the major attractions at Stone Mountain.

■ C L O S E - U P

After parking, return to the sidewalk in front of Confederate Hall and turn left, walking Stone Mountain Loop counterclockwise. Follow the sidewalk 0.2 miles to a trestle for Stone Mountain Railroad. Walk under the trestle and turn left, entering the forest for the first time. At just under 0.4 miles, there is a path to the right, almost hidden in the summer months. Descend a few steps to two polished granite "bridges" across a creek. Return to the main trail and turn left.

Continue on the orange connector trail until a marked right-hand turn at 0.6 miles. This is the entrance to the nature center, which has an interpreted display of plants native to Georgia. Among the trees are mulberry and white oak. Plants include strawberry, Christmas fern, trumpet creeper, fragrant sumac, and beautyberries. As you walk through the garden keep a small building on your left and continue to the other side. Mulberry trees and a railed bridge at 0.7 miles indicate the end of the nature center.

After crossing a stream, the footpath bears right, coming to an intersection with Cherokee (Red) Trail. Turn right and continue to the remains of a house at 1 mile. You can see the roofline cut in the chimney about two-thirds of the way to the top. There are wire cuts in a tree on the opposite site of the house as well. The path bears right at 1.3 miles, climbs a set of railroad-tie steps, and crosses Robert E. Lee Boulevard. Keep a green-fenced playground on your right as you reenter the forest. The trail circles the playground, turning left on a gravel road, then crossing the dam that forms Howell Lake. Step down into the cement overflow, then climb up a similar step on the other side. As the path bears left, there is a railed bridge crossing over a strong creek at 1.5 miles. Just 0.1 mile later, the path crosses Stonewall Jackson Drive.

Venable Lake, on your left, is named for Sam Venable, who ran the quarry early in the 20th century. About halfway around the lake, the trail bears right, crosses a beautiful stream with cascades flowing over a series of large rocks, and then bears left to return to the lakeshore. At 2.5 miles the footpath makes a hard right turn, crossing an earthen dam and turning right on the far side of the lake. On your right is the largest body of water in the park, Stone Mountain Lake.

Just before 2.8 miles, Stone Mountain Loop rises around a rock outcropping, turns inland, makes a right just before the road, and falls to a creek. The trail becomes undefined crossing granite outcroppings, but watch for white blazes on the rock. The number of trails to the lakeshore increase, and the covered bridge comes into view at 3.2 miles. W. W. King built the lattice bridge in 1891. Originally, the bridge spanned the Oconee River in Athens, but when the Georgia Department of Transportation replaced the bridge in 1965, they offered it to Stone Mountain Park for $1. The park accepted the offer and moved the bridge to its present site at a cost of $18,000.

The footpath falls to the lakeshore and crosses an outflow on two granite tablets. The path runs adjacent to the lake, inches above the water level and with a granite wall on the left. Watch for two sets of two granite hearts put in the pathway by an energetic stonemason. As the path curves to the left, away from the lake, concrete walkways replace the trail at 3.6 miles. The network of walkways offers views of the Stone Mountain gristmill, but head for the millwheel and a boardwalk that runs next to the mill for a close-up look at the structure. At the far end of the boardwalk, turn right and continue uphill to a granite sluice and springhouse. Keeping the sluice on your right, cross a field and small stream, turn left, and climb to Robert E. Lee Boulevard.

After you cross the road, the trail winds its way through second-growth forest, mostly oak and beech, then climbs railroad-tie steps to cross the tracks at 4 miles. A nature garden established by the Atlanta branch of the National League of American Pen Women in 1961 is on the left. After you pass under the alpine-style Skylift cables, keep a small garage at 4.4 miles on your right as you circle to the right and climb to Memorial Plaza.

As the path curves to the left, it turns to Chattahoochee stone, and the carving comes into view for the first time.

The massive relief sculpture of Jefferson Davis, Robert E. Lee, and Stonewall Jackson is carved in the world's largest piece of solid rock and represents the work of three sculptors over a period of 56 years. Gutzon Borglum began working on a concept for the sculpture in 1916, although actual carving did not begin until 1923. He quickly ran into problems, first with his system to project the carving onto the mountain, then with just about everybody involved in the project. He left Georgia just ahead of a police car. Next came Augustus Lukeman, who gave up on Borglum's original concept and blasted it off the face of the mountain. Lukeman had made significant progress on the current carving when the project failed to meet its deadline in 1928. The partially completed carving sat for 30 years at the intersection of two rural highways.

When the state of Georgia purchased the land in 1958, it immediately set out to complete the work, hiring sculptor Walker Hancock—although Roy Faulkner, who had no previous experience carving stone, did most of the work. Dedicated in 1970, the project was completed in 1972. On the right, across a field, is Memorial Hall, containing an excellent museum that highlights the mountain, the sculptors, and some local history.

Stone Mountain Loop turns left, crosses railroad tracks, and bears right, reentering the forest. At 4.5 miles the railroad depot is on the right, on the far side of some picnic tables and the tracks. It is a re-creation of the Atlanta depot that Sherman destroyed in his 1864 March to the Sea. General admission tickets allow access to all attractions. Because of seasonal and hourly variations, check **www.stonemountainpark.com** for current pricing information. Behind the depot is the recently added Crossroads, an area of shops designed to resemble a frontier village, with areas called the Treehouses and the Great Barn, and a 4-D theater with a film about the Southern art of storytelling.

Past the picnic tables, the trail runs between the mountain and the railroad and continues in a shortleaf and loblolly pine forest on a frequently rocky trail, occasionally moving into full sun when it climbs on solid granite outcroppings of the mountain. The red-blazed Cherokee Trail heads off to the right at the marked intersection at 5.2 miles, then Stone Mountain Loop runs adjacent to the tracks as it crosses a paved road and enters the Confederate Hall complex.

■ TO THE TRAILHEAD

Take I-285 East to Exit 39B, Stone Mountain Freeway East (Snellville, Athens) and drive 7.8 miles to the exit for Stone Mountain East Gate. The road curves right, then comes to a gate. After the gate, this road is known as Jefferson Davis Drive. Continue 1 mile to where the road splits. Bear left and merge onto Robert E. Lee Boulevard. Follow it 1 mile to Confederate Hall. Turn left and park.

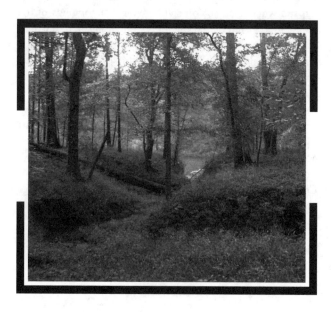

Atlanta South

15 Starrs Mill Trail

■ OVERVIEW

LENGTH: 1.5 miles	**MAPS:** USGS Senoia
CONFIGURATION: Out-and-back	**FACILITIES:** None
SCENERY: Red mill and dam, river views	**SPECIAL COMMENTS:** No bodily contact with the water allowed. The mill is occasionally used as a filming location for movies and local TV. It was featured in *Sweet Home Alabama*, a 2002 film starring Reese Witherspoon. The dark red mill with a white porch and white trim was the glassworks shop where Josh Lucas's character also served food.
EXPOSURE: Full sun	
TRAFFIC: Light	
TRAIL SURFACE: Gravel road	
HIKING TIME: 45 minutes	
ACCESS: October–March: daily, 6:30 a.m.–6 p.m.; April–September: daily, 6:30 a.m.–8:30 p.m.	

■ SNAPSHOT

Explore Starrs Mill, the pond that powers the mill, and Whitewater Creek, and view a swamp at the north end of Starrs Mill Pond.

■ CLOSE-UP

Starrs Mill is the picturesque centerpiece of this 16-acre Fayette County Park. Purchased by the county water system in February 1991, the park contains both Starrs Mill and Starrs Mill Pond, which the county intends to use as a water source as demand increases.

From the small gravel parking lot, walk toward the mill. Before the steps to the porch, there is a ramp made of concrete blocks. Follow this down to Whitewater Creek, below the dam. When water levels are low, a small shoal extends almost entirely across the creek and affords a good place to see both the dam and the mill. Return to the mill's porch steps from the shoal. Built on

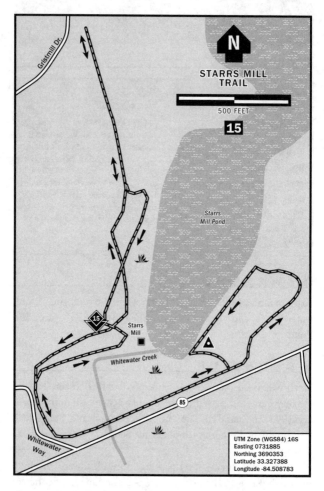

aboveground pilings, the millworks were housed underneath the mill, but the grinding was done in the mill itself. A door on the river side of the mill allowed access to the millworks.

Many years ago, mills such as this were the focal point in rural areas nationwide. Farmers would bring their grains to be ground (or cracked: hence, the term cracker). Mills were places to exchange political views and gossip and normally included a post office or small grocery. Many times, towns would spring up around mills, as did the town of Starrs Mill.

Be careful climbing the steps to the mill's porch—even a casual inspection shows signs of rot. As you reach the top of the stairs, peek inside the window for a look at the grinding apparatus in the center of the floor. Continue on and exit down the front of the porch, returning to the gravel road. Past the mill is an outbuilding, around which the road curves as it rises. Once around the building, follow the road to a T-intersection and turn left.

On your right is an extensive marshland that makes up the upper reaches of Starrs Mill Pond. In the distance you'll probably see at least a few of the larger common swamp birds, including egrets, herons, and mourning doves. As the road begins to rise, a "No Trespassing" sign indicates the park boundary. Turn around and return to the T-intersection, then continue straight ahead. As the road curves to the right, it returns to the lakeshore.

Fishing is a popular pastime at this pond, and anglers normally park at least a couple of cars along the road. The clear land at the water's edge offers an excellent view of the entire lake. During late fall and early spring, migratory birds, especially geese, visit the pond. Return via the gravel road to Starrs Mill parking lot. From the lot walk past the picnic tables down to the river's edge and follow it, walking away from the mill.

Looking down Whitewater Creek, notice the luxuriant growth along the banks. These vegetated borders are known as the riparian zones, and the full, lush growth is indicative of both a healthy river and clean water. The plants hold the banks in place, even during high water, and provide nesting grounds for amphibians and insects and shelter for small animals. As you walk along the river it suddenly makes a 90-degree turn and flows toward the bridge over GA 85. At this long-distance view, notice that the creek's riparian zones continue as far as the eye can see.

Return to the gravel road and follow it as it curves to the left to the entrance of the park at Waterfall Way. Turn left, continue to GA 85, and turn left again. Walk over the bridge across Whitewater Creek and turn left down a dirt driveway.

Continue walking along the creek side, toward the dam. After heavy rainfalls the size of the water flow over the dam enhances photographs of the mill. Once past the dam, you'll see the lake, and on windless days the mill reflects in the millpond. Photographers should get here before sunrise to capture the mill in the morning light. Mid-November is especially beautiful, thanks to the autumn colors of the maple trees behind the mill.

As you walk along the lakeshore, the path reaches the low rise that forms the swamp and becomes overgrown. Turn right and continue to the road embankment, then turn right again and return to the gravel driveway. Climb to GA 85, turn right, and return to the parking lot via Waterfall Way.

■ MORE FUN

Dauset Trails in Jackson features hiking, biking, and horseback trails. It is open Monday through Saturday from 9 a.m. to 5 p.m., and Sunday from noon to 5 p.m. Call (770) 775-6798 for more information.

■ TO THE TRAILHEAD

From Atlanta take I-85 South to Exit 41, Moreland/Newnan. Turn right on Alternate US 27 and travel 0.4 miles to GA 16. Turn right and travel 15.3 miles to GA 74. Turn left on GA 74/85 and continue for 3 miles. At a traffic light, GA 74 turns left. Continue straight ahead on GA 85. Continue 0.3 miles after the light and turn left at Whitewater Way (gravel road). Turn right at 0.1 mile to enter the park.

■ OVERVIEW

LENGTH: 3 miles	**USGS Palmetto**
CONFIGURATION: Loop	**FACILITIES:** Restrooms, picnic tables at the entrance to the park; restrooms at the nature center
SCENERY: 3 separate falls, large rock outcroppings and boulders	
EXPOSURE: Full sun until you cross Bear Creek, then mostly shaded	**SPECIAL COMMENTS:** Learn all about the history of the area, and its natural history, and view an assortment of animals at Cochran Mill Nature Center, through which the trail passes. There are separate trails for mountain-bike enthusiasts and equestrians. The Nature Center is open Monday through Saturday, 9 a.m. to 3 p.m.
TRAFFIC: Heavy to Bear Creek, moderate to the falls, then light	
TRAIL SURFACE: Compacted dirt, portions on rock outcrops	
HIKING TIME: 2 hours	
ACCESS: Open year-round, dawn–dusk	
MAPS: At Cochran Mill Nature Center, a privately run facility adjacent to the park;	

■ SNAPSHOT

After crossing Little Bear Creek, the trail follows an old road to Bear Creek, where it climbs along the riverbank to two falls. From the second falls, it rises to an old road and explores the Bear Creek watershed.

■ CLOSE-UP

Cochran Mill is one of those great hikes full of unexpected bonuses. Owen Henry Cochran inherited his father's land near Bear Creek and for many years ran a water-powered gristmill that his father had built. His brothers expanded the operation around the start of the 20th century. With the coming of electricity to rural Georgia, water power was no longer desirable, and the mill was abandoned. In the 1940s the land was used by the Klan for unknown purposes. Unfortunately, both mills were burned, and the dam to create the millrace was partially

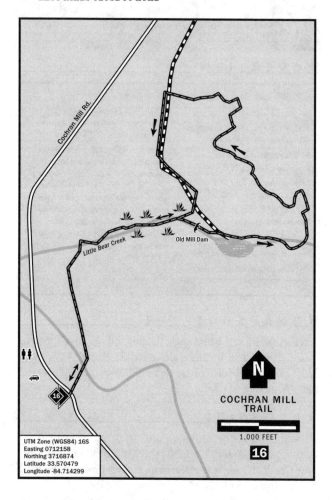

destroyed by vandals. A 48-foot-wide fieldstone dam built by Owen's brother remains. Fulton County built facilities on the 800-acre site, and in 1985 the privately funded Cochran Mill Nature Center was built beside the park.

From the parking lot, cross Cochran Mill Road, then follow the gravel road as it curves left and begins a moderate descent to Little Bear Creek. A concrete bridge has been sealed off to prevent people from using it, but carefully step down to the creek on the left side of the bridge. This is one we cross barefoot because it is deep and wide, ensuring wet feet.

As you cross the creek, watch on the right for the first of three falls along the hike. Put your shoes back on when you get to the far side of the creek because the grass is hard on bare feet. At the top of the hill near the bridge you'll have additional scenic views of the falls. From the bridge, travel straight ahead and down a level gravel road that takes you into a diverse hardwood forest. At 0.3 miles you'll find wild strawberries at the base of a large rock outcropping on the right. When the road comes to a fork 0.1 mile ahead, take the road on the right and continue to a second bridge, this one over Bear Creek. A cleverly arranged entrance is designed to be wide enough for a human but too narrow for bikes and horses. After crossing the bridge, turn right and begin to climb in full shade at an easy-to-moderate grade along the bank of Bear Creek.

If you watch closely, you will see an old yellow blaze every once in a while, but don't worry if you don't see it. Except in a couple of places on rock outcroppings, the trail is well worn and easy to follow. One of these rock outcroppings comes quickly at 0.7 miles into the hike. Keep the river and falls on your right and climb until the trail enters the woods, still near the stream's bank. As you reenter the full shade of the forest, there is an area of perma-mud. At 0.8 miles the trail splits; bear right—the other path is the return from the loop. Following the split the footpath begins to make a significant moderate climb.

Watch for the destroyed dam on the right; water emerges on the left, falls a few feet, and slides back to the right. Not much else remains of Owen Cochran's mill. As you climb the rock outcropping, you will see a large stone with a square center cutout. It marks the path, which rises to a level road with an embankment on the left. Still following the creek, the trail begins to curve left at 1.2 miles. At the curve, watch for an excellent view of wetlands in the distance.

Climbing into the watershed of Bear Creek on a moderate grade, you'll reach the top of an unnamed knoll. The trail then falls to a small creek, which it crosses on a wooden plank bridge with no railings. After the bridge the trail bears right and begins to climb the next knoll. Just before the top, the path makes a left-hand turn, then descends to Cochran Mills Nature Center. Entering from the back, you will pass a large iguana and other animals before coming to the wooden building. We stopped and talked with Rick McCarthy and Cory Washington, who were very helpful, especially with area history, and we got to spend time with some unique creatures.

With the pond on your right, walk along a gravel road to a trailhead kiosk off the road on the left. Follow the path as it descends to a left turn at 2.1 miles. About 0.2 miles later, bear right at a three-way intersection and continue to the right when the trail crosses a stone outcrop returning you to the middle falls of Bear Creek on your left. Continue along this trail to your car.

■ MORE FUN

From mid-April to the first week in June, the Georgia Renaissance Festival allows visitors to experience Renaissance Europe. Performers such as the Tortuga Twins and the Zucchini Brothers (Ripe and Green) entertain the masses until it's time for the jousts. The event is held weekends, including Memorial Day, from 10:30 a.m. to 6 p.m.

■ TO THE TRAILHEAD

Take I-85 South to Exit 56, Collingsworth Road (Palmetto/Tyrone). At the end of the ramp, turn right on Collingsworth Road. At 0.1 mile Collingsworth goes straight as Weldon Road heads off to the left. Collingsworth becomes Fayetteville Road. At a four-way stop at 2.4 miles, turn right on Toombs Street. Turn right on Hutchinson Ferry Road at 0.3 miles. Travel 1.4 miles and turn right on Cochran Mill Road. Travel 4.1 miles to the parking area on the left. Cochran Mill Nature Center is ahead on the right.

 Ocmulgee River Trail

■ OVERVIEW

LENGTH: 5.2 miles	**HIKING TIME:** 2 hours
CONFIGURATION: Out-and-back	**ACCESS:** Open year-round
SCENERY: Ocmulgee River floodplain, some good views of the Ocmulgee River	**MAPS:** USGS Berner
	FACILITIES: None
EXPOSURE: Some sun	**SPECIAL COMMENTS:** The footpath now continues to the Ocmulgee River bluffs, about 16 miles from the trailhead.
TRAFFIC: Light	
TRAIL SURFACE: Packed dirt	

■ SNAPSHOT

The trail parallels the Ocmulgee River along its floodplain, occasionally moving inland to circumvent a tributary or marshy area.

■ CLOSE-UP

Ocmulgee, meaning bubbling water or boiling water, is the name that was given to this strong, wide river by the Hitchiti tribe. Early British explorers knew it as the Ocheese Creek and called the native people living along the river near present-day Macon the Creek. The Hitchiti was one nation within the Creek Confederacy. It is believed, but cannot be proven, that the Creek were the descendants of Mound Builders who built cities near the

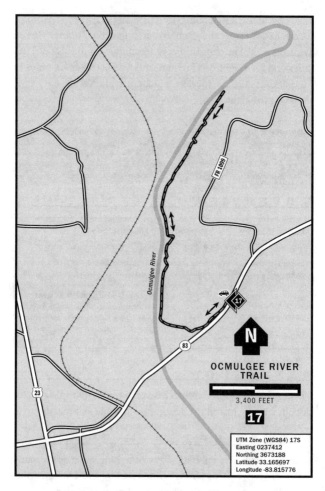

OCMULGEE RIVER
TRAIL

3,400 FEET

17

UTM Zone (WGS84) 17S
Easting 0237412
Northing 3673188
Latitude 33.165697
Longitude -83.815776

confluence of two or more rivers throughout Georgia. Ocmulgee, Etowah, and Kolomoki mounds are all examples of the work
of America's first tribal civilization in Georgia.

As we pulled into the Oconee National Forest parking
area, a family of wild turkeys hurried away from the rear of the

parking area, so watch out for wildlife throughout the hike. Ocmulgee River Trail begins by rising through the forest and quickly beginning an easy, even descent toward the river on a wide, roadlike path. Throughout most of the hike, the trail is wide, narrowing occasionally to cross a stream or swampy area, making this a good family hike. After dropping 200 feet in 0.6 miles, the trail reaches the Ocmulgee River and easily curves to the right to parallel the wide, fast-flowing watercourse. Throughout the hike the Ocmulgee will be on your left on the way out, and on your right on the way back. Car noise quickly disappears as you walk away from GA 83 along the riverbank. From here on, watch carefully for poison ivy.

You occasionally have long-distance views from the trail, and there are oaks and elms along the path. Many of the elms are large and have deep furrows and ashen-gray bark, indicating they are fairly old. These elm trees, along with substantial oaks, anchor the healthy riparian zones on either side of the river. The U.S. Forest Service, which manages the area, permits horseback riding on the trail. During our hike we noticed evidence of horses and spotted a number of fairly common birds and wildlife, including wood ducks, vireos, squirrels, deer, and raccoons. Since the river is along their migration path, large numbers of waterfowl can be spotted during the spring and fall.

As the trail comes to the first tributary of the Ocmulgee, it bears right (inland), making a wet-foot crossing of a stream at just under 1 mile. The trail climbs away from the river again at 1.2 miles, crossing a wooden bridge without rails, and climbs to a primitive camping area at 1.3 miles. You can walk through the camping area to a small, forest-service parking area or simply make a hard left at the start of the primitive camping area. On the trail's return to the Ocmulgee the river traverses a swampy area before climbing to the riverbank 0.1 mile later. From here the trail follows the riverbank closely, only occasionally dropping into the lightly forested floodplain. At 2.6 miles the trail turns inland to cross another stream. Although we could see that the trail continues, this looked like a good place to turn around and head back to the car.

■ MORE FUN

The Ocmulgee River flows south to Macon, where it passes through the Ocmulgee National Monument, an Early Mississippian Mound Builder site that flourished between 900 and 1150 AD. Within the park grounds are a museum and several larger mounds that are fun to climb. To get there, return to I-75 South and take Exit 165; follow the signs to I-16. Take Exit 2 and turn left on Coliseum Drive. In 0.6 miles turn right on Emery Highway. Follow this road 0.8 miles. The entrance is on the right.

■ TO THE TRAILHEAD

Take I-75 South from Atlanta to Exit 187 (GA 83/Forsyth/Montecello). Turn left on SR 83, known locally as North Lee Street and Cabaniss Road. The highway crosses US 23 and begins a descent to the Ocmulgee River. After crossing the river on a double bridge, the road begins to rise. Watch on the left for an unmarked pulloff big enough for five or six cars. The trailhead is on the river side of the parking lot, near the highway, on top of a small mound.

18 Panola Mountain Trail

OVERVIEW

LENGTH: 3.3 miles (including a 1-mile fitness path)	**ACCESS:** Open year-round, $4 park entrance fee
CONFIGURATION: Double loop	**MAPS:** Interpreted trail maps are available at the trailhead kiosk; USGS Stockbridge, Redan
SCENERY: Some good long-distance views from rock outcropping	
EXPOSURE: Much of the trail is in full sun.	**FACILITIES:** Natural history exhibits, interpreted trails, restrooms
TRAFFIC: Moderate, especially on weekends	**SPECIAL COMMENTS:** A ranger-led hike on the third Saturday of the month explores environmentally sensitive Panola Mountain. Call beforehand to be certain the hike is scheduled and to reserve a spot.
TRAIL SURFACE: Mostly dirt but some stone	
HIKING TIME: 1.5 hours	

SNAPSHOT

Two interpreted loop trails take hikers though two very different environments; the first trail drops to a creek that is occasionally dry, while the second climbs one of Panola Mountain's many outcroppings.

CLOSE-UP

Panola Mountain State Conservation Park was established in 1971 and is Georgia's first conservation park. Located on a massive granite rock outcrop, its job is to protect many of the environmentally sensitive areas within the park, both biologic and geologic, on this 100-acre monadnock (single mountain). The trails within the park are individual loops, and the only developed side trails take visitors to interpreted areas. The trails involve less than a 150-foot elevation change, with the greatest part of that on Watershed Trail.

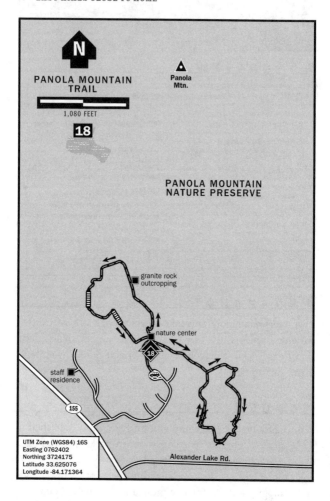

First stop by the nature center and pick up two pamphlets, one for Watershed Trail and one for Rock Outcrop Trail. Exiting the nature center, continue to a large trailhead sign and turn right. After passing through a pine blowdown with evidence of a fire, Watershed Trail begins an easy descent as it enters a fertile piedmont lowlands with hickory, oak, and sumac. The trail is wide and strewn with wood chips, but it changes to a dirt trail as it drops at an easy grade to a three-way intersection. Continue straight ahead, in the direction the pamphlet describes, to reach a creek. Watch for streams that carry watershed runoff down to the creek, shaping the landscape as they go—the path crosses two of these on bridges. The first station leaves the trail to take hikers to a small gully created by erosion.

Stations 2 and 3 continue the hydrology lesson, but Station 4 takes hikers out to a flat "pavement rock" formed by an exfoliation process enhanced by the creek water. Finally, the interpretive stations introduce hikers to lichen, a plant that grows on exposed granite to create an environment where some plants, especially red moss, may follow. Cross another bridge and begin climbing back into the watershed of the stream. As the loop trail comes to a T-intersection at 0.8 miles, turn right and return to the trailhead.

At the trailhead, turn right again and follow Rock Outcrop Trail. This trail traverses a vastly different environment than Watershed Trail, and circles a low hill with surprising drops off to the right and a thicker forest to the left. The tree mix has also changed, with loblolly pine, sweetgum, black cherry, and hawthorn accenting white oak on this yellow-blazed trail. The trail begins to descend when you see the first of the massive granite outcrops at 1.2 miles. Less than 0.1 mile later, this hike passes rock cairns; a single pole rail keeps visitors on the proper path. Because of the sensitive environment, please stay on the hiking trail and don't be tempted to stray. If you would like to spend time on similar slabs, see Stone Mountain Loop (page 68). A small portion of the trail does traverse the granite.

After viewing the granite, continue to two boardwalks—one to the right, the other to the left—that take you to the trail interpretation. There is a small outdoor theater on the left before you reach the trailhead kiosk.

If you decide to make the ranger-led trek to Panola Mountain, be certain to wear comfortable hiking shoes. The loop hike travels 3.5 miles to the largest exposed granite slab in the park and back again, and you'll stop frequently to discuss various topics.

■ MORE FUN

Continue south on GA 155 to McDonough, turn left on John Frank Ward Boulevard, then turn right on Lemon Street and proceed to GA 81. Turn left on Lake Dow Road and enter Heritage Park. Baseball fields occupy most of the park, but it does have a 0.9-mile multiuse track and a heritage area that's worth a visit. The park is open from 8 a.m. until 11 p.m. and features a covered bridge and a veteran's memorial. A visit to the Heritage Museum requires you to make an appointment; phone (770) 288-8421.

■ TO THE TRAILHEAD

From Atlanta, take I-20 East to Exit 68, Wesley Chapel Road. Turn right and, at 0.3 miles, turn left at a traffic light, onto Snapfinger Road. The entrance to the park is 5.8 miles on the left. Continue to the end of the road; enter the nature center.

19 Piedmont National Wildlife Refuge Trails

■ OVERVIEW

LENGTH: 3.8 miles	**HIKING TIME:** 2 hours
CONFIGURATION: Double loop	**ACCESS:** Open year-round
SCENERY: Lakeside and creekside views and forested wetlands	**MAPS:** Available at trailhead kiosk; USGS Dames Ferry
EXPOSURE: Full sun in the vicinity of Allison Lake and the dam; mostly sunny on Red-Cockaded Woodpecker Trail; mostly shaded on Allison Lake Trail, except near the lakeshore	**FACILITIES:** Visitor center on the road is open Monday–Friday, 8 a.m.–5 p.m.
TRAFFIC: Light	**SPECIAL COMMENTS:** This is an excellent trail for bird-watchers and wildlife lovers, but be wary of ticks and chiggers.
TRAIL SURFACE: Compacted dirt trails, gravel roads	

■ SNAPSHOT

This hike combines Red-Cockaded Woodpecker Trail and Allison Lake Trail to take you through a wilderness rich with wildlife.

■ CLOSE-UP

Our introduction to the Piedmont National Wildlife Refuge was certainly thrilling. A black vulture with a wingspan as wide as the road led us to the trailhead, finally rising above the tree line and turning away from Allison Lake. Ringed in fieldstone with a dark-brown roof, the trailhead kiosk contains extensive information on the creation and goals of Piedmont NWR and the National Wildlife Refuge Program in general. You'll also find information on the preservation of species native to the park, including the endangered red-cockaded woodpecker.

In 1939 President Franklin D. Roosevelt created Piedmont NWR by executive order. The land was substantially different at

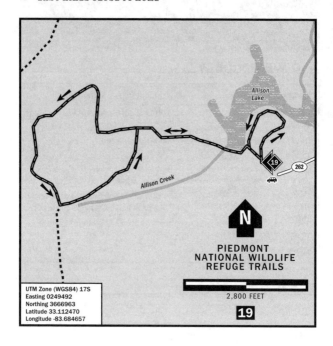

Allison Lake

Allison Creek

N

PIEDMONT
NATIONAL WILDLIFE
REFUGE TRAILS

2,800 FEET

19

UTM Zone (WGS84) 17S
Easting 0249492
Northing 3666963
Latitude 33.112470
Longitude -83.684657

the time than it now appears. Cleared and planted by settlers who grew cotton as their cash crop, the land was mostly abandoned by 1939 because of decreasing cotton prices, boll-weevil infestations, and the Great Depression. The biggest problem facing the newly created refuge was erosion—the land was almost completely barren.

Today, thanks to more than 60 years of effective management by the U.S. Fish & Wildlife Service, and Mother Nature, the refuge is returning to a more natural state. The symbol of this regeneration is the red-cockaded woodpecker. The "red" in the bird's name refers to a small patch of color on either side of the bird's head that appears during mating season and territorial battles. The woodpecker is black and white with a large white cheek surrounded by a black head cap and nape on either side of its head.

Both Red-Cockaded Woodpecker (RCW) Trail and Allison Lake Trail begin behind the kiosk. The RCW heads off to the left, making an easy descent through the woods to a gravel road. Turn right and continue descending to a well-marked left turn at Allison Lake, where the trail enters full sun and begins to cross the earthen dam that forms the lake. In the center of the dam, slanted cement sides lead to a flat, wide spillway that you have to cross, but may make the trail impassable after a heavy rain when the spillway has running water. Continue on the gravel road to the marked entrance to RCW Trail on the left at 0.3 miles.

Almost immediately you enter a typical southeastern shortleaf pine second-growth forest that is one of the woodpecker's habitats. Although this bird prefers mature pines infected with red-heart fungus, it can be attracted to healthy, younger-growth trees with a little help. The Wildlife Service produces habitats by using artificial inserts, essentially creating a cavity in the pine. The birds nest in these cavities carved in living trees; you'll easily spot the nests by the sap running from them. It is believed that the woodpeckers use the sap to defend against predators, such as the rat snake. Trees with inserts are marked with a white circle at the base.

A wooden bench at 0.6 miles marks the start of the loop trail. Turn right and begin a descent to a wooden bridge over a small creek. After the creek the trail bears right and rises to a small knob. On sunny summer days, the area has a number of butterflies, including the tiger swallowtail, viceroy, and zebra. At 1 mile, after the footpath curves left, a gravel road heads off to the right. Just past the road, the trail begins climbing to its highest point.

Begin an extended easy downhill over the next 0.6 miles. Just after beginning the descent, you'll reach a large field with a widely spread group of pines, clearly marked at the base with a ring of white paint. The cavities created by the Wildlife Service attract the woodpeckers and creatures that compete with them for similar nesting, such as the nocturnal flying squirrel. Just past the field, a rarely used road joins the path on the right.

As the trail begins to parallel a creek, the descent eases. Just before you cross the normally dry creek, watch for a red maple with evidence of yellow-bellied sapsuckers. In addition to the maple, this area of hardwoods includes tulip poplar, sweetgum, and a variety of oak. Finally, at 1.8 miles, the trail reaches Allison Creek and a forested wetland that appeared to be fairly active. As the trail began its climb back to the start of the loop, we noted an active beaver den. The trail also lost its definition, but follow the "well-worn trail" principle to return to the bench where the loop started, at 2.3 miles. Turn right and return to the trailhead kiosk.

On the fall day on which we visited Piedmont Wildlife Refuge, the Allison Lake Trail was packed with all kinds of animals, from common to exotic. Bring your binoculars and be prepared to spend some quiet time in a blind when walking this trail that begins behind the trailhead kiosk to the right. The trail is interpreted, so pick up a brochure at the kiosk. The numbers in the brochure correspond to those on signs bearing symbols resembling a hiker's boot print. Unlike RCW Trail, the Allison Lake Trail is mostly shaded, except for a portion by the lakeshore. At the start, shortleaf pines dominate, but as the trail descends the knob, the number of hardwoods increases.

Initially, the pathway descends, crossing a number of normally dry creek beds, then it rises to a knob. A flash of yellow in the pines led us to believe a pine warbler was out looking for insects. Descending the knob, the trail falls to the lake, eventually turning left and running parallel to but above the lakeshore. On the far side of the water, we spotted deer and wild turkey that were surprisingly close to one another. The plaintive call of the mourning dove and the rat-a-tat-tat of a woodpecker added to the excitement.

Finally, on the approach to the lake, we realized we were in for a treat. A kingfisher watched the water for fish. On the far side of the shore, a snowy egret waded among the grass, not bothering a line of turtles sunning on a submerged branch. At 3.4 miles a blind for watching waterfowl juts out into Allison Lake.

■ MORE FUN

The Whistle Stop Cafe in Juliette, Georgia, is well known for its fried green tomatoes. It was featured in the film *Fried Green Tomatoes* starring Jessica Tandy and Kathy Bates in 1991; phone (478) 994-3670. Jarrell Plantation is a Georgia State Park featuring an interpreted tour of an 18th-century Georgia estate. The plantation is open Tuesday through Saturday from 9 a.m. to 5 p.m., and Sunday from 2 p.m. to 5:30 p.m., but is closed Mondays (except holidays) and on Thanksgiving, December 25, and January 1. Also, it is closed Tuesday when it's open on Monday. Phone (478) 986-5172 for more information.

■ TO THE TRAILHEAD

Take I-75 South to Exit 186, Juliette Road/Tift College Drive. Turn left on Juliette Road, at the end of the ramp. After crossing a bridge and passing through East Juliette, the road becomes Juliette-Round Oak Road. At 11.8 miles bear left at the Piedmont NWR sign. (The road to the right goes to Jarrell Plantation.) In 5.3 miles turn left on a paved road (designated GA 262 on maps but not on the road). After 0.8 miles the road to the visitor center bears right, and the road to the left continues to the trailhead at 1.3 miles.

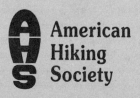